Advance Praise for
Yoga: The Poetry of the Body

"Rodney's long-awaited book is finally here! The poetry of yoga is expressly evident within these pages, and the conversational tone lends interesting insight into the mind of one of the world's most popular yogis. This book will be read for years to come."

—ERICH SCHIFFMANN, AUTHOR OF
YOGA: THE SPIRIT AND PRACTICE OF MOVING INTO STILLNESS

"Rodney Yee has created a unique and masterful book on yoga. Like Rodney himself, *Yoga: The Poetry of the Body* is playful, practical, and personal. It combines instruction, dialogue, and philosophy to create a feast of inspiration and insight."

—PATRICIA WALDEN, INTERNATIONAL YOGA TEACHER AND
INSTRUCTOR FEATURED IN BESTSELLING YOGA VIDEOS BY GAIAM

"Thank you, Rodney and Nina, for a beautiful and poetic guide into the happy, radiant spaces of yoga practice. The instructions are clear and metaphorical. They give a feeling of what it's like to really be there at peace with the vibrance and depth of the body and mind. I highly recommend this book for both total beginners and advanced students of yoga!"

—RICHARD FREEMAN,
INTERNATIONALLY ACCLAIMED ASHTANGA YOGA INSTRUCTOR

yoga

The Poetry of the Body

RODNEY YEE

WITH NINA ZOLOTOW

Photographs by Michal Venera

THOMAS DUNNE BOOKS

St. Martin's Griffin New York

THOMAS DUNNE BOOKS.
An imprint of St. Martin's Press.

www.stmartins.com

Book design by Kathryn Parise

Photographs by Michal Venera,
courtesy of Rodney Yee and Nina Zolotow

Hair and makeup by Helen Jeffers

Permissions appear on page 337.

LIBRARY OF CONGRESS CATALOGING-IN-PUBLICATION DATA
Yee, Rodney.
Yoga : the poetry of the body / Rodney Yee with Nina Zolotow.—1st ed.
p.   cm.
Includes bibliographical references and index.
ISBN 0-312-27331-2
1. Yoga, Haòha.   I. Zolotow, Nina.   II. Title.

RA781.7.Y44 2002
613.7'046—dc21   2001054496

First Edition: January 2002

10 9 8 7 6 5 4 3 2 1

Contents

Acknowledgments

We used to wonder sometimes when we saw long acknowledgment pages that went on and on thanking all kinds of people "without whom this book wouldn't be possible." I mean, who even knows that many people, much less needs them all just to write a book? But now here we are eating crow, because it turns out that quite a number of people besides us did a lot of work on this book, and most of them for nothing more than the fun of it.

The following people reviewed parts or all of this book: Vickie Russell Bell, Richard Koman, Rebecca Lemov, Leza Lowitz, Rosemary O'Connor, Dirk van Nouhuys, Melitta Rorty, Richard Rosen, Ian Swensen, and Carol Williams. Thank you all. Your suggestions helped us clarify our ideas and enriched the book, while your enthusiasm kept us going during times of doubt (will anybody but us, we wondered, find these dialogues at all interesting?). By the way, Dirk, you win the prize for editing the largest number of pages—almost the entire book. How about lunch sometime soon?

The following people tested the yoga practices for us: Baxter Bell, Anja Borgstrom, Rebecca Lemov, Melitta Rorty, and Ian Swensen. Thanks to all of you for letting us know what worked and what didn't work in actual practice.

Richard Rosen helped us with the Sanskrit and English names for the yoga poses. Thank you, Richard, for your time and your expertise.

Lisa Olsen Stewart obtained the permissions for reprinting the various poems in our book and also helped out with a myriad of small administrative tasks. Lisa, you have been invaluable.

Then there were the photo shoots . . .

Edith and Milton Zolotow helped us with the basic layout of the book and with the art direction of the photographs. Thank you for your graphic design expertise and for the simple, elegant style of our yoga photographs.

Donna Fone, Rodney's wife, organized the photo shoots and was our female model, giving her time unstintingly. Special thanks to you, Donna, both for your management skills and for your beautiful yoga.

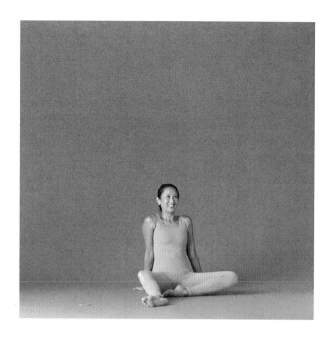

Athena Pappas also assisted with the primary photo shoot. Thank you so much, Athena, for your yoga expertise and for giving us an entire weekend.

Thank you, John Hall and Elnora Lee of Color 2000 in San Francisco, for your wisdom and your photographic support, thank you, K.D.dids, for the yogawear Rod wore for the cover shot, and thank you, Yoga Mats, for the props used in the interior photos.

Evan, Adesha, and Johanna Yee, and Rosie and Quinn Gibson did not actually do any work on the book, but they're our kids and everyone always mentions their kids in the acknowledgments (besides, Quinn did have to eat vegan food for an *entire* week at one of Rod's yoga retreats just so we could finish our first draft on time).

Finally, Rod wants to say to Donna, "One more thing you have seen me through. Let's take a vacation now." And to Professor Bradford Wayne Gibson, Nina wants to say, "Thank you, darling, for being the bad guy of the book. It was an ugly job, but someone had to do it."

About Rodney Yee

Rodney Yee—I didn't even want to study yoga with him in the first place. I'd heard that his classes were completely packed—fifty students jammed, mat to mat, into a relatively small studio—and that he wasn't even there half the time, what with the workshops and retreats he conducts all over the United States and abroad. Furthermore, with all those yoga videos—how many are there now? seventeen?—and magazine articles, I thought he must be really full of himself. But my friend Melitta finally dragged me to Hawaii to one of his yoga retreats saying, "Nina, you *have* to come"—and it was immediately obvious that here was a great teacher.

When you take a class from Rodney Yee, the first thing you notice is the passion with which he teaches. His tremendous energy and just plain joy sweep you along so that two hours of a demanding physical "workout" become an all-absorbing, inspiring experience. He's been teaching yoga locally and worldwide for over fifteen years, day after day, so where does all that excitement come from? I believe the wellspring is simply the deep love he has for yoga, for both the physical art and the underlying philosophy. For he fell in love with yoga more than twenty years ago, after his very first class. As a twenty-three-year-old ballet dancer and ex-gymnast, he had gone to yoga class in the hope of becoming more flexible. Instead he discovered a practice that satisfied him in a way that neither ballet nor gymnastics had ever done—body and soul. And his commitment to that practice, as well as to his teaching, has only deepened as the years have passed.

Then you listen to his clear instructions and mull over the individual corrections he addresses to you and to other students. (To me he says, "Lead with your heart, Nina, not your head," and tells me to spend part of every day in a passive back bend with my shoulder blades—ouch—draped over a wood block; and he tells Melitta, who has a strong, muscular runner's body, "Soften your work, and see if you can align and support yourself more on your skeletal structure and less with muscular determination—try being more playful.") And you soon become aware of his profound understanding of the body. Of course, Rodney's a very well trained yoga teacher, who was certified by the Iyengar Institute of San Francisco and who pursued additional studies with the Iyengars in India. And his formal training along with twenty years of personal practice have given him a solid base of technical knowledge. But he's also someone who was born with a great natural gift for reading and understanding bodies of all kinds, just as someone is born with a talent for music or the visual arts. Even before he became a yogi, he was always fascinated by the human body. As a small child, he stared with wonder at kids who could sit with their legs bent backward as if they were broken (in Hero Pose, as yogis call it), while he, with his tighter body, could not. Why was that? This led him to interests in gymnastics and ballet, as well as college-level studies in physical therapy, and a lifelong fascination with how much we express with our bodies and what they say about who we are.

Finally, you become aware of the aspect of Rodney that the writer in me loves the most: his unique way with words. Rodney has long felt that poetry is the most accurate way to describe the human experience, and while he is teaching, he uses metaphors, repetition, and other poetic devices to invoke the physical and emotional sensations of yoga. "Let your upper chest flutter with the beat of your heart," he says, "like a baby bird just out of its shell, beginning to unwrap its wings from the sticky glue of its own birth." Sometimes, on one of his more inspired days—of course, they're not always inspired—Rodney striding around his classroom reminds me of Rumi, the famous Sufi poet, who composed all his poetry spontaneously, while whirling round and round a pole in the center of a courtyard.

As I got to know Rodney outside of class, I learned about his interest in philosophy—both Eastern and Western—and his passion for inquiry into the nature of human existence. Do we need to have beliefs? What are we scared of? What is

freedom? Are we ever connected at all—is communication even possible? Is there any difference between the mind and body? What is consciousness? Is there anything beyond our illusions? It sometimes seems as if he can talk about these issues forever—talk and listen both, that is, for he's as full of questions as he is of answers.

So as one of Rodney's regular students at Piedmont Yoga Studio (which I became eventually—he even complains sometimes about the fact that it took me so long), it was clear to me that there were some special qualities about him as a teacher and a yogi that were not coming through in his videos or in magazine interviews. And when he asked me to write this book with him—his first yoga book—I realized that one of the most valuable things I could do would be to capture some of the excitement of what it's like to be present in his classroom, or as Richard Rosen, a fellow yoga teacher and old friend of Rodney's, put it: "bring out the 'Rodness' of Rodney."

In the beginning I wasn't sure of the best way to go about that, so I tried a lot of different things. I sat through his classes and wrote down everything that struck me as particularly "Rod." I took his classes—beginning to advanced—and scribbled down quick notes in between poses. I sat on the floor of his yoga room with my pad of paper while he practiced, and had him talk to me while he did all the poses in this book. And I taped hours and hours of our conversations, and put some of the highlights from those tapes directly into the book. As a result, I give you the Rodney Yee I know in everyday life, or what Rod himself calls "Rodney Yee real-time—live backstage and live onstage, but never staged."

(By the way, his classes *are* really crowded, and he *isn't* there half the time, and sometimes I *still* think he is really full of himself.)

—NINA ZOLOTOW

About Nina Zolotow (and Me)

When I think of Nina Zolotow, the first thing that comes to my mind is a curly-haired woman walking to the grocery store, pulling a red wagon behind her and looking at the world slightly defiantly because she's doing something she believes in. She's walking—and not taking the car—both as a statement and because that's the way she wants to live. To her, this is being human—to walk to the grocery store and get your groceries and put them in a little red wagon and bring them home again. And it doesn't feel as human to have to get in your car, or to live far away from the necessary things in your life, or have your life be convoluted and dampened by the "conveniences" we consider to be modern life. So Nina is a woman who is in search of meaning, but meaning in everyday things.

I first knew Nina as a yoga student. But even in just the way she approached the practice, I saw an earnestness in her—an earnestness to be intrigued by the complexity of the body—and a certain determination that was something like: If you're willing to be here digging away, I'm willing to be here digging away, too. And it's not so much

that we're going to find anything profound, but maybe just the digging itself has its own profundity. She's been interested in yoga for a long time. She studied for a couple of years before the birth of her first child, and then, after a long break, she took it up again about eight years ago. However, it's only been in the last four years that she's been practicing intensively and developing her home practice.

Later on, when I got to know Nina personally, I learned that she had left her longtime career as a technical writer to pursue her interest in creative writing, which was something I really admired. And when she let me read some of her one-sentence stories (a few of which are in this book), I was excited about them because in a very short amount of time they evoked a strong emotion in me, something that has always been an important aspect of art for me. I also felt that this was someone who was doing in writing what I'm trying to do in my yoga practice and in my teaching. (What I mean by that is that I've never been interested in teaching a yoga class that's purely about technique—even though I could easily do that. It's much more important for me to use my mechanical understanding to unearth the emotional content.) So immediately I thought, maybe this is the person I need to write with.

I do think, however, that Nina's background in technical writing aided her in writing this book. Her skill in writing instructional manuals not only helped her organize the book and write simple, clear instructions, but it enabled her to force me to be more accurate with words, to keep the information in the book accessible to beginning students, and to stay on schedule. I also think that twenty years as a technical writer helped her in getting out of the way in some sense, to allow me to find *my* voice. In the beginning of our collaboration, I wasn't sure how this was going to work —would having two people write together mean that we ended up with just another impersonal technical book? But Nina's ability to get out of the way when necessary—to stand back even though the book was about something she really cared about—allowed us to create a book that feels really personal to me. There is a lot of me in the book and a lot of her in the book, and then there are the parts that we crack up about at this point—the parts that are both Nina and me at the same time, maybe even mixed together in a single sentence. But the last time I read this book, I was struck by the fact that during all those hours in which we had sat face-to-face, Nina had really heard what I had to say. This collaboration makes me feel that the division between two minds does have a bridge: Much of this book is where our minds have met. And that is one of the most fulfilling parts of yoga, when one mind dissolves into another.

—RODNEY YEE

About This Book

Are you wondering if yoga is for you? Well, maybe it is. Because everyone can do yoga. You can be male or female, young or old, flexible or stiff, well or sick, healthy or injured. And we hope this book will help you decide whether you want to make yoga a part of your life.

A lot of people are scared of yoga because they've seen someone doing weird-looking positions and they think, oh, I can't do yoga because I'm so inflexible. And they may be intrigued, but they think that yoga is so far from their body vocabulary that they decide, why even try? But doing yoga doesn't mean that you have to go beyond what you can already do. You can just play with the range of motion that you have. For within any limitations, you have infinite possibilities.

Yes, a lot of people think that they have to be healthy to do yoga. But the point is to use your body as it is at the present moment, whether your lower back hurts, you just broke a leg, or you're a well-tuned athlete. Just use all the sensations—the sensation of well-being, the sensation of pain, the sensation of sickness—to make an inquiry into your body, breath, and psyche. Who are

you? What are your dreams? What are your fears? What is your story? What do you really want?

Basically, the only thing that matters is that you are alive, that you are curious about who you are—your body, your mind, and your emotions—and that you are willing to play with and enjoy the gifts that you've been given. Of course, you should use your common sense. If you are injured, don't ignore your injury by being aggressive or complacent. But the yoga poses in this book are the most basic of yoga poses. And the most important thing is for you to listen, really listen, to what your body is telling you.

Here's what you can do. Start by simply reading the book, from beginning to end. Then set aside twenty to thirty minutes, take off your shoes and socks, and do the first yoga practice in the book, A Playful Practice. After that, do each of the practices in Part 3, in the order in which they appear. Do the practices whenever you can find the time, one each day for a week, one a week for a couple of months—whatever you can manage. If you have any questions or just want to know more about an individual pose as it comes up in a practice, you can check the detailed information on the poses in Part 5. Part 5 contains every pose that appears in the practices in Part 3.

If you are interested in exploring your breath, you can do the breath exercises in Part 4 in addition to the yoga postures. See Part 4 for information on when and how often to practice.

In some ways the yoga practice is very simple. It allows you to do movements and body positions that are very natural and yet not common to our vocabulary and in our present-day society. And in doing these movements and postures that our everyday life does not call for, we begin to get a sense of freedom in our bodies. Our bodies get to move the way they want to move. Our feet get to be out of shoes and socks and feel the ground. Our arms get to reach above our heads and extend in all directions, in front of us and beside us and in back of us. Our spines get to flex and extend and twist. Our hips get to rotate and feel circular movements in their sockets. And just these very simple, natural combinations of movements can begin to unlock our natural desire to be free in our bodies and to be free in our minds.

This book contains a lot of different kinds of things: yoga practices, yoga poses, and breath exercises, as well as photographs, conversations, poems, and one-sentence stories. We've designed this book so you can either work through it sequentially or just wander through it. It is a journey into yoga that will introduce you to some of the myriad possibilities that yoga provides for moving and playing, and for allowing new ideas to spring forth.

If I feel physically as if the top of my head were taken off,

I know that is poetry.

—EMILY DICKINSON

PART 1

Why

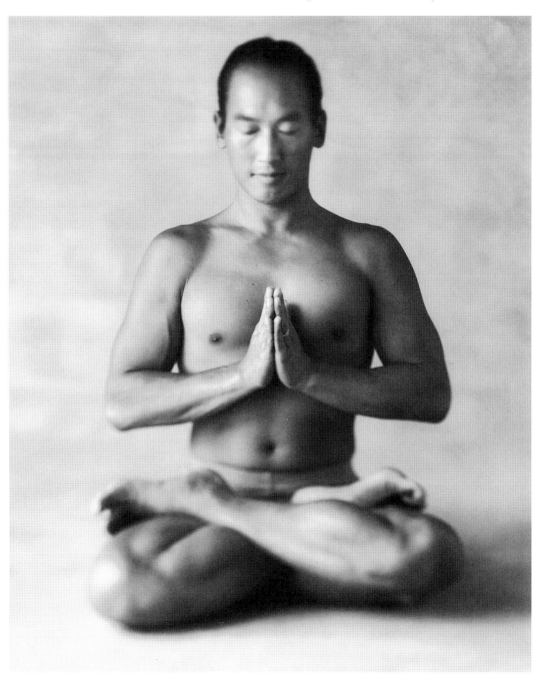

A COAT

I made my song a coat
Covered with embroideries
Out of old mythologies
From heel to throat;
But the fools caught it,
Wore it in the world's eyes
As though they'd wrought it.
Song, let them take it,
For there's more enterprise
In walking naked.

—WILLIAM BUTLER YEATS

Why We Do Yoga

ROD   So you're practicing now, and it feels like maybe it's a part of your life. You're pretty busy—you're a mom, you have a partner in life, you're doing a lot of other work, you're writing, obviously. When do you fit it in, usually, during the day?

NINA   Well, right now I have more free time than I used to because I'm working on a book, and so I do practice in the afternoons, most days. But I started practicing regularly while I had a full-time job. So I began by doing my yoga in the evening after my children were in bed, at about eight-thirty at night. And I took class three times a week—I had a midday class in my office building—so that helped. But I definitely get—then and now—constrained by my life and my family commitments.

ROD   It sounds like you have a number of obstacles; in fact, probably all the familiar obstacles anybody has to doing this practice. What made you practice? What got you there? What made you go past the obstacles?

NINA   I think it was because I wanted to be stronger. And I felt like if I could do certain yoga poses physically—be physically flexible or strong—I could be that way emotionally, too. I wanted to learn handstand, back bend, and push-up position because I wanted to be stronger—

ROD   So now you can do handstand—I've seen it. You can do a back bend. Your back bends are actually quite good. You can do push-up position in Sun Salutations. So has that worked? Has it made you stronger? Do you feel elated? Do you feel like some of your goals have been achieved?

NINA   Yes, I do. I feel stronger physically, and it makes me—I don't know that I feel stronger emotionally, but I feel more confident.

ROD   *Confident* is not stronger emotionally?

NINA   There's a certain part of me that still feels really fragile—

ROD   Well, why wouldn't someone want to feel fragile? I think fragility is one of the most underrated things as a human being. I believe that we're doing yoga so that we can be strong enough to be fragile. I mean, we *are* fragile, and we're living in a society where we could easily be destroyed—psychologically, emotionally, and physically—so why shouldn't we feel fragile? Life is on a silk thread hanging like a cocoon from a tree, and it's a fragile thing. I don't think yoga is to keep you from feeling fragile. I think it's to enable you to be consciously fragile but still feel like, "I'm fine with this fragility."

PART 2

Before You Practice

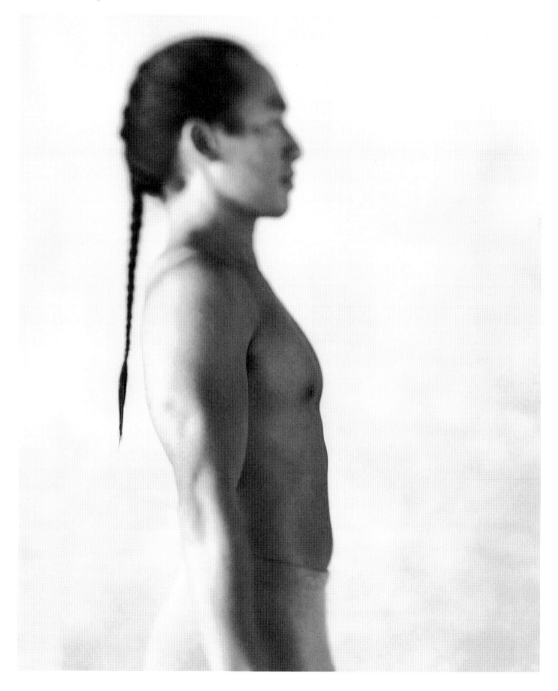

CREMATION

It nearly cancels my fear of death,
    my dearest said,
When I think of cremation. To rot in
    the earth
Is a loathsome end, but to roar up in
    flame—besides, I am used to it.
I have flamed with love or fury so
    often in my life,
No wonder my body is tired, no
    wonder it is dying.
We had great joy of my body. Scatter
    the ashes.

—ROBINSON JEFFERS

Getting Ready to Practice

It would be wonderful to be able to say that all you need to do yoga is your body. And to a certain extent this is true, because you *can* do yoga almost anywhere—at the beach, in a hotel room, in an office cubicle, or even in an airplane. However, a few inexpensive yoga props (such as a folded blanket or a wooden block) can make such a big difference to your practice that we recommend using them at times. And wearing the right clothes can make a difference, too, because certain types of tight clothing, such as jeans, can restrict your ability to move. So this section provides basic information about all the equipment you need to start a yoga practice:

- your body (and your mind)
- yoga clothes
- props

About Your Body (and Your Mind)

The most important pieces of equipment you need for doing yoga are your body and your mind. Your body is your tool for living, the instru-

ment through which the music of life is played. But how well do you know it?

When you start to do yoga, whether from a book or a video, or in a class, you begin to work with individual parts of your body that you may never have tried to move before or whose names you might not even know. So we would like you to take some time before you begin the practices in Part 3 to look at and feel your body, and to learn the basic "body vocabulary" that we will be using throughout this book.

Remember being a kid and getting a tool kit or a lab set for Christmas—how you unwrapped and opened the box and then sat looking at its contents with wonder: what are all these things for?

Your Feet

Sit on the ground in a simple crossed-legged position, as shown in the photograph, on the next page, and take one of your feet into your hands. First, massage your foot (that's always a good thing). Then specifically massage the following:

- ball of your foot
- your big toe mound

- your heel, including the back, middle, front, and sides of your heel
- the arch of your foot (both inner and outer arch)
- your Achilles tendon

Your Legs

Sit in Staff Pose, as shown in the photograph, and lightly massage the following:

- shin
- calf
- front of your thigh
- hamstring

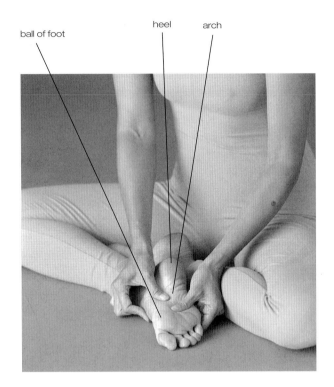

ball of foot   heel   arch

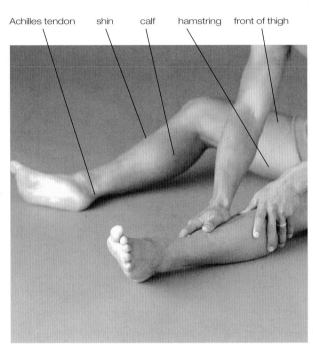

Achilles tendon   shin   calf   hamstring   front of thigh

Inward and Outward Rotation. Next, still in Staff Pose, bend your knees and watch your legs as you turn your feet in (big toes toward each other) and out (big toes away from each other), then in and out again. As your feet and legs rotate inward and outward, look at your feet, look at your knees, and look at your thighs.

Now straighten your legs again and repeat the same actions with your feet, turning them in and then out. Again, as your feet and legs rotate inward and outward, look at your feet, look at your knees, and look at your thighs.

The position of your knees and thighs that occurs when you turn your feet in is called *inward rotation*. The position of your knees and thighs that occurs when you turn your feet out is called *outward rotation*.

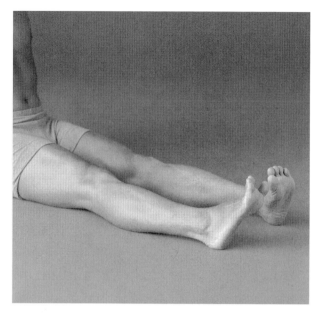

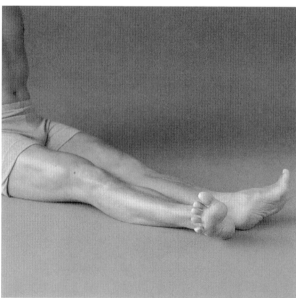

The Back of Your Pelvis

Sit on your heels, as shown in the photographs here (if you can't sit on your heels, place a folded blanket on top of your heels and sit on that).

Reach your hands under your buttocks to feel your *sitting bones*, and then move your hands up to feel the tops of your buttocks by your lower back. Then use your hands to find the top of your *sacrum* and follow it down to your *tailbone*.

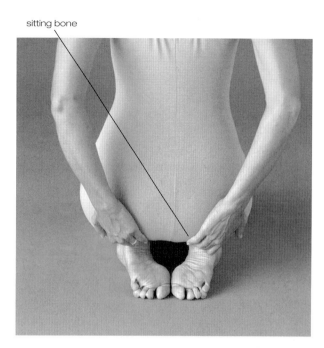

sitting bone

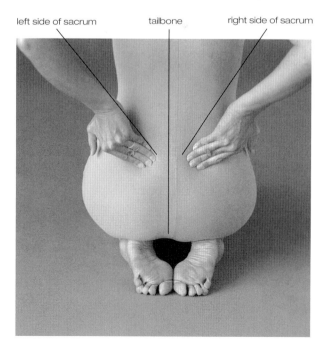

left side of sacrum   tailbone   right side of sacrum

The Front of Your Pelvis

Sit in Cobbler's Pose, as shown in the photograph. Now slide the outer edge of your hands down your *groins,* moving your hands from the *top* of your groins toward the *bottom* of your groins, near your genitals. (People always ask, "Where are my groins?" Well, your groins are the narrow valleys where your inner thighs meet your pelvis.)

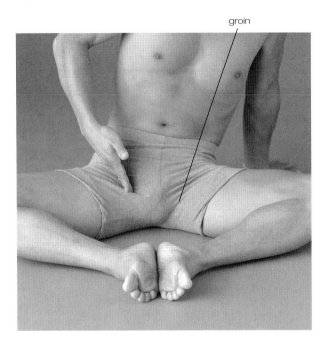

Deepening Your Groins. Next sit in a simple crossed-legged position. Now rock the top of your pelvis back and forward, and observe your groins. As you lean back and rock the top of your pelvis back, your groins will get *shallower.* As you lean forward and rock the top of your pelvis forward, your groins will get *deeper.* In this book, when we tell you to *deepen* your groins, we mean for you to relax your groins downward so the valleys get deeper, rather than letting them flare open.

Your Front Body

Lie on your back with your knees bent and the soles of your feet on the ground, as shown in the photograph. Now lightly touch your front body in the following places, feeling the soft parts and the bony ones:

- groins
- hip point
- belly
- solar plexus
- lower ribs

- middle ribs
- upper ribs
- sternum
- collarbones

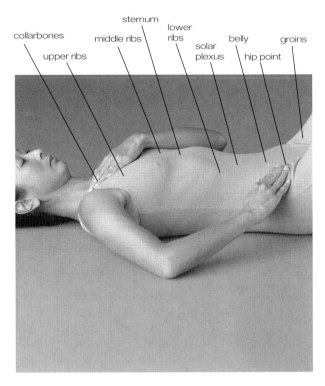

Your Back Body

Fold a single blanket into quarters, and roll it into a tight single roll. Then lie on your back, as shown in the photograph. The rolled blanket will help bring your awareness to various parts of your back body, parts you usually don't see or think about.

1. Position the blanket roll under your neck, and bring your awareness to the *back of your neck* and its natural curve.
2. Move the blanket roll under your shoulder

blades. Then move your arms around, and bring your awareness to your *shoulder blades* and *upper back*.

3. Move the blanket roll under your middle back, and bring your awareness to your *back lower ribs*.

4. Move the blanket roll under your lower back, and bring your awareness to your *lumbar region* and the *natural curve* of your lower back.

5. Move the blanket roll under your sacrum, and bring your awareness to the *sacrum* and *tailbone*.

6. Move the blanket roll under your thighs, and bring your awareness to your *hamstrings*.

7. Move the blanket roll under your lower legs, and bring your awareness to your *calves*.

- armpit-chest
- back of your skull
- crown of your head
- temples

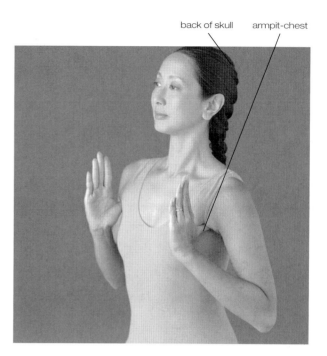

back of skull   armpit-chest

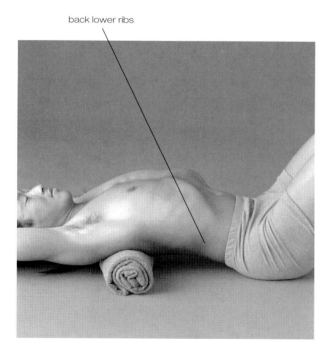

back lower ribs

Your Chest, Neck, and Head

Take a basic standing position, as shown in the photograph, and gently touch the following parts of your body:

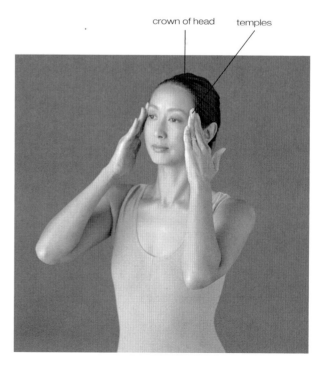

crown of head   temples

Your Mind

While you were exploring all those areas of your body, where was your mind?

Try looking at your hand for a few moments. Gaze at the back of your hand, and then turn it over and gaze at your palm. Observe it in all its details, in all its beautiful complexity. Be amazed, like a baby noticing its hand for the first time. Does your mind tend to wander? Does it bother you that your mind wanders? Can your mind be in your body?

Next try to observe your breath for a few moments. Notice the outer sensations—the rise and fall of your chest, solar plexus, belly, and back. Notice the inner sensations—your inhalations as they enter your body and your exhalations as they leave it. What is the difference between concentrating on something in the present moment and on something that is just in your head? *Is* there a difference?

Ask yourself: when I am watching my mind, what is watching my mind?

About Yoga Clothes

Don't worry—we're not going to tell you that you need to buy a bunch of new stuff. It's just that what you wear while you do yoga can influence your ability to move freely and to find your balance. While it is true that there is a lot of specially designed "yoga wear" available from specialty catalogs and yoga studios, we're pretty sure you can put together something suitable from things you have around the house.

Bare Feet

The most important thing to wear while doing yoga is bare feet. And by *bare feet*, we mean com-

pletely naked feet—so do not wear shoes of any kind (we've seen people trying to do yoga in aerobics shoes) and no socks or stockings or tights with feet on them. Bare feet not only keep you from slipping around on the floor, but they bring you into direct contact with the ground, renewing your connection to the earth and allowing you to find your balance with much greater sensitivity.

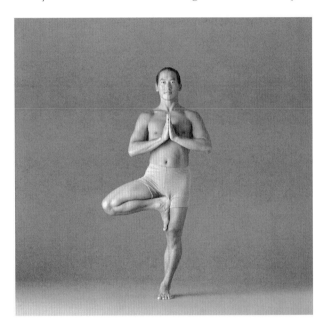

Clothes That Allow You to Move

Many of the other yoga books we've read say to wear "loose, comfortable clothing," but while we agree with the comfortable part, we wonder about the loose part. The main point is that you should not wear clothes that restrict your ability to move, such as tight jeans or a tailored dress shirt. However, loose clothing, such as big T-shirts and baggy sweatpants, can get in your way when you are doing yoga (like in Downward-Facing Dog; a big T-shirt slides down your body and falls right into your face, which gets really annoying after a while).

So Rodney simply tells you to wear as little as possible. He even says, "Do yoga in your underwear." That way there will be nothing to get in your way and you can see the subtle movements of your body. Besides, bare skin on skin is best for doing Tree Pose and other poses where one part of your body rests on another part of your body (no sliding around on slippery fabric).

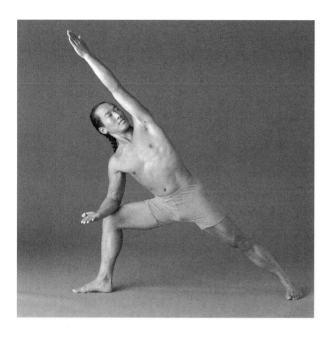

Of course, you might not be ready for this, and besides, sometimes it gets cold. So see if you can find any of the following in your dresser drawers:

- gym shorts or boxer shorts
- bicycle shorts
- leggings
- tank tops or muscle shirts
- fitted T-shirts
- sports bras
- leotards

When you're doing restorative poses (as in A Relaxation Practice on page 148), you may start to cool down, so you can pull on a sweatshirt or sweater over your yoga clothes. For Relaxation Pose (see Part 5), feel free to lie under a warm blanket (and you can even put your socks back on for this one).

About Yoga Props

Why Do I Need Props, Anyway? Props enable you to achieve a more natural alignment so you can deepen your pose by paying attention to the subtle aspects of the pose (not just to screaming or burning muscles). They also allow you to stay in the poses longer so you can feel some of their deeper effects. Sometimes a prop even changes the entire feeling of the pose, such as in Legs Up the Wall Pose (page 314). With a bolster, Legs Up the Wall Pose opens your chest and your heart, freeing up your breath. Without the bolster, Legs Up the Wall Pose provides great, equal support for your back but does not open your chest. Many of the photographs in the eight yoga practices in Part 3 show the poses with props. And many of the individual pose descriptions in Part 5 include a modification of the basic pose that uses one or more props.

When Should I Use Props? As you practice, it is a good idea to try the same poses both with and without the recommended props. If you are new to yoga, try using the props the first time, and then experiment without them. If you are an experienced practitioner who has always done the poses without props, try using props for a change. As always, use your yoga practice as an opportunity to question and change your habits, to play and explore and learn. Ask yourself: how does this prop (or lack of it) affect my body, my mind, my emotions?

What Do I Really Need? What we're going to do here is present the ideal list of props you should have for doing the poses and practices in this book. (You can get yoga props from most yoga studios, and you can also order them from specialty catalogs by mail or on the Web. See Appendix A for information.) However, because we know you're probably not going to run out and buy all this stuff immediately, we'll tell you how to fake certain yoga props using things you probably already have in the house.

1 yoga mat (aka sticky mat). Description: a thin, sticky rectangular rubber mat, with dimensions of ⅛ × 24 × 68 inches.

The purpose of a yoga mat is to keep you from slipping around on the floor or rug. If you buy just one prop, let it be a yoga mat. But if you don't have a yoga mat, do *not* use a cushy exercise mat, a camping pad, or a futon, and no, not your bed, either. It is difficult to balance on a cushy surface, and it is better to be right on the floor or on a dense carpet if you don't have a sticky mat (no shag carpets, though—they're too spongy).

1 yoga block. Description: a block of wood or foam, with dimensions of 4 × 6 × 9 inches.

The purpose of a yoga block is to provide a solid raised surface on which you can sit or rest your hand or fingers. If you do not have a yoga block, you can use a hardback book wrapped with tape so that it doesn't fall open and has an even surface on the ends.

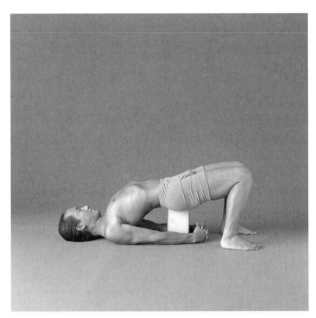

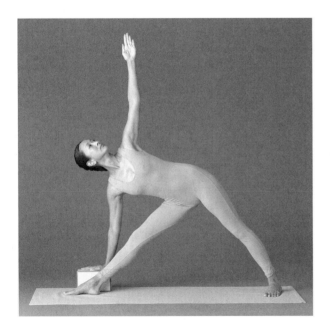

1 yoga belt (aka yoga strap). Description: a specially designed cotton belt with a buckle, with dimensions of 1½ inches × 6 feet.

The purpose of the yoga belt is to allow you to reach one part of your body (such as your toes) that you normally can't reach with ease. If you do not have a yoga belt, check your closet for any soft cloth belt or tie (what about the belt on your bathrobe?).

2 blankets. Description: a single-size blanket of dense wool or cotton, with dimensions of approximately 62 × 80 inches.

The purpose of a blanket—usually folded into a rectangle—is to provide a firm raised surface on which you can sit or over which you can drape your body. There are official yoga blankets available for sale, but any single-size blanket will do, as long as it is of thick, densely woven material, such as wool or cotton (no fluffy quilts or comforters, please, or thin thermal blankets because they're too spongy).

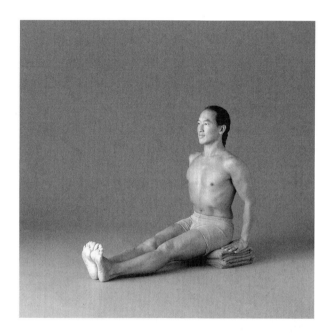

1 round bolster. Description: a specially designed firm cylindrical pillow available from specialty catalogs.

The purpose of a round bolster is to provide a firm rounded surface over which you can drape your body. If you do not have a round bolster, you can fake one by folding and then rolling one or two blankets (see The Art of Blanket Folding on the next page).

1 flat bolster. Description: a specially designed firm rectangular pillow available from specialty catalogs.

The purpose of a flat bolster is to provide a firm rectangular surface on which you can prop up your body or over which you can drape it. If you do not have a flat bolster, you can fake one by folding and then stacking two blankets (see The Art of Blanket Folding on the next page).

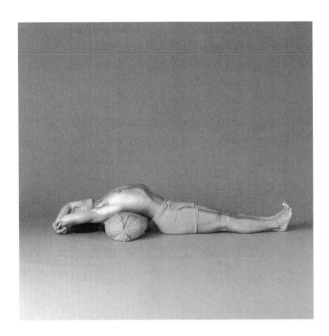

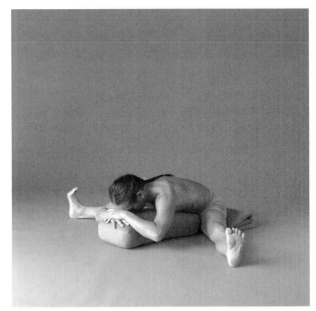

1 eye pillow. Description: a small rectangular cloth bag filled with flax seeds, with dimensions of approximately 1 × 4 × 8½ inches.

The purpose of an eye pillow is to cover your eyes during Relaxation Pose and other restorative poses, which helps to relax your eyes and your face. An eye pillow is by no means a necessary prop, but some of us think they are heavenly, especially the ones scented with lavender. If you do not have an eye pillow and you want to cover your eyes during restorative poses, you can use a folded washcloth or silk scarf.

The Art of Blanket Folding

Be sure to approach your first experiences with blanket folding in a spirit of patience and mindfulness. In other words, slow down and fold your blankets carefully. It is actually important for you to have neat, precisely folded blankets. A neatly folded blanket provides an even, symmetrical surface that your body can understand and rest on. But a sloppy, unevenly folded blanket can throw your body out of alignment, making it worse than not using a prop at all.

Basic Rectangular Fold. The first step in mastering the art of blanket folding is to learn to fold a single blanket three times into a basic rectangle of approximately 31 by 20 inches. This basic rectangle is a good size for sitting on as well as the starting point for making a bolster.

To create the basic rectangle:

1. From the short edge of the blanket, fold the complete blanket in half so the two short edges come together into a neat rectangle (approximately 62 × 40 inches).
2. From the short edge of this rectangle, fold the blanket in half again so the two short edges come together in a smaller rectangle (approximately 31 × 40 inches).
3. From the short edge of this rectangle, fold the blanket in half again so the two short edges come together into a smaller rectangle (approximately 31 × 20 inches).

Creating a Round Bolster. Depending on the thickness you want, you can create a round bolster by using one blanket to make a thinner roll or two blankets to make a thicker one.

To create a single blanket roll:

1. Fold a blanket three times into a neat basic rectangle (as described above).
2. From the short edge of the basic rectangle, roll the blanket into a single tight roll.

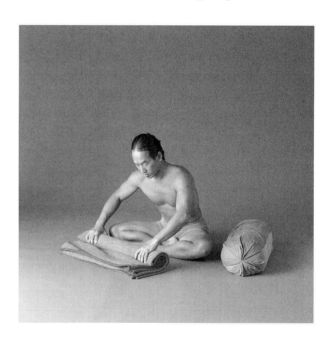

To create a double blanket roll:

1. Create a single tight blanket roll as described above.
2. Take a blanket that you have folded into a single basic rectangle, and place the single blanket roll on top of it, at the short end. Now roll the basic rectangle around the single blanket roll.

Creating a Flat Bolster. To create a flat bolster, you need two blankets that have been folded three times into basic rectangles (as described above).

1. From the long edge of the basic rectangle, fold the first blanket so that the long sides come together into a long, narrow rectangle.
2. Repeat for the second blanket.
3. Now you have two long, narrow rectangles. Stack the two rectangles on top of one another so that their thick folded edges are directly opposite each other.

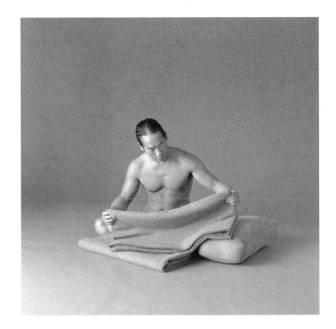

About Body Image

NINA   I'm familiar with some of the issues women have about their bodies, both because I am a woman and because these concerns seem to come up in class. For women, the belly comes up a lot in class because some women feel like they need to have flat bellies, and so to stop sucking in their bellies—to have a soft belly—feels embarrassing or shameful. And a lot of women feel like they shouldn't stick their butts out because they don't want to have big butts—this comes up in class when we're told to release our groins and let the spine take its natural curves. I've never heard anyone talk about breasts in any yoga class, but that's an issue for me—with all the emphasis on chest opening—of feeling uncomfortable with drawing attention to that part of my body. But those three things for me are women's issues: belly, butt, and breasts. I could try to guess what the men's are, but I want to know what you say, because I've never heard anyone talk about those.

ROD   Well, why do you think there are not very many men in yoga class? Because of one big factor, and that is that they think that yoga class is about flexibility, and most men have the image of themselves that they're really quite stiff. But really where they're stiff is in their head.

NINA   [laughing] I hope that tone of voice doesn't come through on paper!

ROD   But that's true. I would say that's the number one reason why most men haven't been in yoga class—because they think that they actually won't be very competent at it.

NINA   Well, you know what? They're not, and they're very unhappy about it. They come into class, and they've been running and weight lifting or whatever, and they think they're strong—I saw this happen all the time in my office building with the guys from the gym. They would come to yoga class and see these women in the front row who had been doing yoga for a while, and the women could do all these things that the men couldn't. And they couldn't handle it. I'm serious! They would leave after a week.

ROD   Well, see, there you go. Men are actually very strongly into body image, even though in some ways their body image comes from the capability of doing a sport rather than from the shape of their body. So that's where yoga intimidates them because, in some sense, their body actually doesn't function very well. And in yoga class you'll put a bunch of men in hand-stand, and they can't hold it very long because their arms are slightly bent, and they're using all muscle and no bone. You put them in Downward-Facing Dog, and they can't hold it very long because there's so much resistance in their hamstrings that it's pulling them out of the pose. And they feel awkward with hip openers and forward bends, usually. And even back bends—their shoulders are usually really stiff. So a lot of men are intimidated by yoga. The funny thing is, of course, for thousands of years yoga was just practiced by men! So we're having a real switch-over here in the United States, which is interesting.

   But let me continue with men and their body images. I have a story about a woman who came up to me in Florida and thanked me profusely for making the yoga for abs [abdominal muscles] video. Because she had been trying to get her husband into yoga for about ten years, to no avail. And then one day, her husband came up to her and said, "Umm . . . honey . . . could I, uh . . . would you mind buying me that tape on yoga for abs?" And so there you have part of men's issues with body image: Even though there are a lot of men walking around with big bellies, this is one of the things they're most self-conscious about—the belly area. How are they going to deal with this middle-age spread—their college pants don't fit them anymore, and their bellies are hanging over their waistlines?

NINA   But yoga isn't about losing weight, is it? It's not about getting rid of middle-age spread or making yourself look younger.

ROD   Yes, one of the most profound effects of yoga is that people start getting comfortable with the body they've been given. More than just wanting to change it all the time, they come to a place of acceptance and even appreciation for the body that they have.

I myself had that experience. I came from a ballet background, and my legs were never long enough and my muscles were never flexible enough. I just basically felt that I was never enough and that something was *wrong* with my body. But after around five years of yoga, I started really liking my body. That was an enormous change for me, and I do attribute that to yoga. Because it wasn't so much what I could do or couldn't do with my body, it was that in looking at my body deeply, and really seeing it and playing with it and having fun with it and being interested in it and being curious about it, I realized it was just a huge playground for fun. A playground for exploration and interest. It was like—wow—my body is a fun thing to explore.

NINA   It's like the article we were reading in the *New York Times*, "Maybe We Are Alone in the Universe." That made me feel—if we're the only planet in the universe with intelligent life, then the body's even more of a miracle. It's already kind of a miracle, but that made it seem even more miraculous.

ROD   Yes, "kind of a miracle." I mean, you ask any scientist—even if the universe is spotted with human life or with intelligent life, still, from any point of view, the ability for the earth to evolve this way, as a place where the human being could have evolved, the chances of that are so slim. So yes, I think it is one thing to know that intellectually, but in yoga you actually begin to know that on a visceral level. You have deep appreciation for what it means to be alive.

NINA   Actually, that's what I do every time I do Relaxation Pose at the end of a practice. I say, "I'm grateful for this chance to practice yoga. And I'm grateful for my wonderful body that lets me do yoga."

ROD   I've witnessed this in people with all different shapes and forms to their body. I feel like they come to this realization through the practice of yoga, and it's a wonderful gift that this practice can unveil.

For example, one of my students told me the other day that she was always the fat girl in PE class. We were talking about humiliation—about different times in our lives when we were humiliated about our bodies. And she just said, "Try being the fat girl in PE class!" Then she went on to say that yoga was the first thing she could do where she felt like she wasn't humiliated for being a large woman, where she actually began to feel good about her body and what it did and what it could do. She said it was really the first time for her that she had that feeling. There was another woman sitting at our table who said she'd also been humiliated in PE class—she'd been literally picked up by the leg and told, "Oh, you can't do this." She's a psychotherapist, and she said that doing yoga made her feel for the first time like her body was something she could be proud of. That can make a big difference psychologically and emotionally.

NINA   In a way we're talking about how yoga makes you more comfortable with your body. But what about the fact that when you're doing yoga, there can be inhibitions that you have about your body that hold you back from being able to do a pose?

ROD   Yes. A lot of people—even in yoga class—may not try a pose or may not do a pose because they think, oh, I'm going to fall out of that, or I'm going to be embarrassed in that. So we still have some of the same tendencies to hold back or not try something because we might be in a humiliating situation.

NINA   [laughs] Like Reclined Cobbler's Pose, the pose where you have to lie with your belly so vulnerable and your groins exposed. To lie in a position like that—

ROD   Yes, that's true. I forget about it since I've been working with the body for so long. We do a lot of postures that make us actually—on a pure animal survival level—very vulnerable. I mean back bends, for instance—your hands and feet are on the ground, you can barely move, and all your vital organs are exposed. You're talking about Reclined Cobbler's Pose, which means lying on your back with your legs dropped open—for a woman that's basically as vulnerable as it gets. And that's the thing: you're asked to be in these vulnerable positions, hopefully in a "safe" environment, but you're asked to be in these positions and begin to deal with them, psychologically, emotionally, and physically. It's like: can you feel secure in a position or a moment that's not secure? In other words, can you keep your center in times of danger or in times of fear or in times of vulnerability? In that sense, yoga is a laboratory for us to experiment with keeping our center— maybe like the old saying "keeping your wits about you"—even in situations where your body almost instinctively wants to cover up.

    And many women, I think, have been—what you said to me before— taught to tuck their butts and hide their breasts. And in yoga, we're asking ourselves to go into those places that maybe we've been socially trained to avoid. We're asking ourselves to go to physical postures that are more exposed, and we're asking, "Well, what's wrong with this?" It's a radical practice in that way. Basically, are you supposed to be ashamed of your body? Are you supposed to—

NINA Yes, you are! I think that's true. In our culture we're taught to be ashamed of, and even hate, our bodies.

ROD And yoga is really trying to liberate us from that shame about our bodies. To love your body is a very important thing—I think the health of your mind *depends* on your being able to love your body. But also, another thing I was going to say is that we've made fun of, for instance, Chinese foot binding—for women who were wealthy and didn't have to work, they'd bind their feet as a symbol of wealth. And everybody always makes fun of that and how tortured it is. But look what we put women in the United States in: high-heeled pumps with really narrow toes.

Face it, beauty is a big deal, and it's a bigger deal for women than for men, in some sense, all throughout history. But let me say this about it: no one can deny that someone looks good when they have a glow about them—when some radiance is coming from someone, when their skin begins to radiate aliveness and there's a presence of being. Their eyes are clear, and there's a sense of their body sort of hanging beautifully. Like when you have beautiful clothes and they hang on the human body so well. It's the same thing—when the human body stands aligned and open, there's something unbelievably appealing about that. When people practice yoga and their alignment gets better, and they start feeling good about themselves, and their skin begins to look good, and just in general there's a sparkle in their eyes . . . That doesn't have to be only from yoga, but it seems like some people who do yoga do carry a certain radiance about them.

And you were talking the other day about being a woman and getting stronger in the arms and feeling more confident from that. You know, people expect men to be strong in the arms. But a lot of men aren't, and it is doubly important for a man to get strong in the arms! Women, in some sense, socially aren't expected to be capable with their arms. Maybe they are in doing things that require a delicate touch, but not with, you know, heavy lifting or being able to lift themselves with their arms. So there are a lot of men, actually, who get a lot of self-confidence from yoga because finally now they can—here's an expression—"pull their own weight." But even more than that, a lot of times men are traditionally more tight, partly just because of their structure. A lot of men have really tight hamstrings. To begin to get their hands close to the ground or even to touch their toes—it's almost the equivalent of a woman doing a handstand for the first time.

NINA That's interesting.

ROD   A man all of a sudden being able to touch his toes is like, "Wow, I can touch my toes now with straight legs!"

NINA   What's the feeling? For a woman, it's "I'm strong!" What is it for a guy who finally touches his toes?

ROD   "Wow—getting flexible!" A lot of people don't think their bodies change, actually; that's the funny thing.

NINA   Oh, they think they're stuck. They're stuck with the body they have.

ROD   That's very much the case! I go to parties all the time and people say, "Oh, you're a yoga teacher. I don't do that because I'm tight." And I'm thinking, well, that's exactly *why* I'm doing it, because I *am* naturally tight. It's this great thing, to feel more fluid in the body. Women—they may actually feel weaker in the body, but they feel more fluid than men do. You might not understand that, but I, for instance, am a really good example of someone who used to be *really* tight. I had fairly good coordination, but I was really tight, and it inhibited my fluidity, my ability to be graceful. As I became more flexible in my joints and in my musculature, I was able to move more gracefully and in a sense with much more coordination. And I can't tell you how *great* that feels. It's like wearing really tight jeans and a tight jacket, and it's fine for a while, but when you take it off it feels like, "Oh, God." It's more comfortable and it's less *restricting*. To unbind the body—just in its musculature—is so *comfortable*.

     So I feel a hundred times more comfortable in my body. I'm forty-three now, and I've never felt this comfortable in my body. Most people think at a certain age, you're going to feel more and more uncomfortable—

NINA   Yes, I was actually going to say something like that, because I started doing yoga seriously in my forties. Most people have this idea that all you can do is sort of "maintain" or "hang on," not that you can actually improve or change. And it's actually very exciting to be able to say, "I've learned to do these things that I could never do before, *ever*." And I feel now, still, it doesn't matter, I can keep moving. It's not going to be over. It's not like if you're not a brilliant physicist by the time you're twenty-one, you never will be. You know how there are all these professions where you peak out, and then it's over, like ice-skating or mathematics. But here, it feels to me like there's no end. I can keep going.

ROD   Well, in fact the practice gets richer and richer. And not just on an athletic level—though even there, in some ways, it does—but on the subtle level of knowing your body, the subtle level of being able to feel, of being able to touch yourself from the inside. You get to listen more and more deeply. It's like anything else. If you listen to music, your ear for music gets more accurate. If you do anything with attention for a long period of time, your sensitivity gets greater. In your yoga, your sensitivity to your own inner feelings, to the movements inside, to your emotions, to the movement of your skin, to the way the light is coming into your eyes—you're actually building up the sensitivity. So in some sense, you're more alive.

PART 3

Falling into Yoga

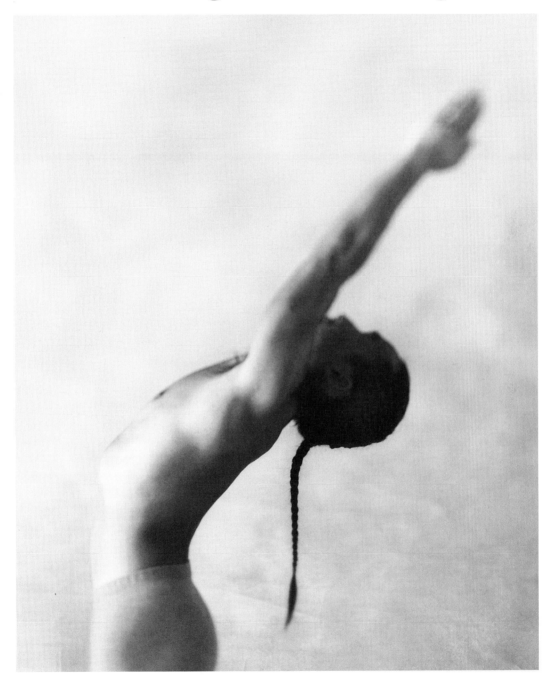

Life is like a cloud of mist
Emerging from a mountain cave
And death
A floating moon
In its celestial course.
If you think too much
About the meaning they may have
You'll be bound forever
Like an ass to a stake.

—MUMON GENSEN

This part of our book is about exploring your mind and your body and the relationship between them. As you do your first yoga postures, your mind will begin to focus on the movements of your body and on the sound and feel of your breath, and you will become aware of their influence on each other.

This is also an inquiry into philosophy and how philosophy translates into action. The themes of the yoga practices presented here compel you to consider how to integrate concepts you have experienced within your body into your daily life, such as playfulness, alignment, relaxation, and resistance. This is self-study—learning about yourself more intimately through the avenue of your body. It is about investigating some of the principles of your physical reality and learning how to question some of the assumptions you make about your physical and mental existence. For instance, what is your habitual posture? And can you shift this orientation and play with it to explore other possibilities?

We ask a simple question: who are you? By watching your body and your breath, you can start to see the deep and subtle movements of your inner body. And begin to dig up treasures from far below the surface of your everyday considerations. We hope these investigations will lead you back into the joy of *not* knowing as you soften into contentment in the heart of mystery.

As you begin to practice yoga, you will observe the nature of your body and your breath and realize that you're constantly falling into the present moment. Then you can begin to relinquish your illusions of control. Your mere acceptance of the state of not knowing unveils your aliveness and drops you into the ever-molting movement of all things. Yoga is this falling. This not knowing. This surrender to the movement of existence.

About the Practices

This part of the book contains a program for "falling" into yoga that consists of eight short yoga practices. We hope that you will do these eight practices in the order in which they are presented, beginning with the Playful Practice and finishing with the Movement Practice.

A Playful Practice comes first because we want to emphasize that your curiosity and your willingness to explore are vital to learning. Can you bring the playfulness you uncover in this first practice with you throughout all your yoga experimentation?

A **Falling Practice** follows because we want you to experience early on that yoga poses are not held but are a constant dialogue in finding center.

A **Grounding Practice** is next because your relationship to the earth is fundamental to all the other practices. The ground is one of your most basic orientations in both your body and your mind.

An **Alignment Practice** builds on the foundation of the Grounding Practice. As you move from the earth upward to construct a myriad of yoga postures, play with their natural, organic alignment.

A **Breath Practice** brings together the architecture of your body and the focus of your mind to the freedom of your breath. It will bring awareness to the more subtle bindings of your body.

A **Resistance Practice** allows you to confront explicitly the mental and physical resistances that arise during any yoga practice. Which poses are you most resistant to?

A **Relaxation Practice** leads you to an understanding of relaxation that will enable you to bring elements of relaxation to all your yoga postures, even the most demanding and active poses.

A **Movement Practice** provides a chance for you to integrate what you've learned from all the other practices into movement. Moving from pose to pose allows you to focus on all your movements, both within the poses and within the transitions that link them.

After you have tried all these practices once in the order in which they are presented, feel free to go back and repeat any of them in any order you wish, any number of times. There will always be more to discover.

Note that for each pose within these practices, we provide only a single photograph and a very brief description. The descriptions are intentionally brief because we want you just to *do* the poses and not to worry about getting them "right." (See the dialogue No Right Conversations, in which we talk about this concept.) However, if at any time while you are practicing, you wish to learn more about a given pose, you can look it up in Part 5: Posing and Reposing. Part 5 contains more photographs and detailed information about each of the poses in Part 3.

About Timing

Counting Your Breaths. To enable you to adapt these practices to your physical capabilities as well as to the free time that you have available, we provide a time range for each pose, with a minimum and maximum number of breaths. We ask you to count your breaths rather than seconds because this allows you to focus inside more easily. Eventually, when you have gained experience with doing the poses for an interval, you can begin to use your intuition to time yourself rather than counting your breaths.

However, if your breath in a particular pose feels too erratic to count, you can use a timer or second hand to time yourself. In this book, we consider six breaths equal to approximately thirty seconds.

The first time you do the practices, we recommend that you sweep through the sequence of poses, staying in each pose for only the minimum number of breaths. After that, you can extend the length of any practice and explore the poses more deeply by staying in the poses for longer periods of time.

Falling Asleep. In restorative poses, such as Reclined Cobbler's Pose (page 312), it is important to set a timer in case you fall asleep. Even though you are trying to slowly build up the amount of time you spend in restorative poses, there is a limit to what is healthy. Therefore, do not stay in restorative poses for indefinite amounts of time. You can even set a timer to go off at specific intervals, such as once every minute, to remind you to bring your consciousness back to the pose.

Asymmetrical Poses. Many yoga poses are asymmetrical, and you must do them two times, first on the right side and then on the left. For these poses, always do both sides for the same amount of time. For example, if you do Triangle Pose to the right for ten breaths, do it on the left for ten breaths as well.

Repetitions. For some poses, we provide the option of repetitions (for example, one to three times). This allows you to explore some of the poses more deeply and also reveals to you how repeating the poses will open them up.

For an asymmetrical pose, doing the pose once means first doing it to the right and then doing it to the left. To repeat the pose a second time, do it again to the right and then again to the left (rather than doing it twice to the right and then twice to the left).

For back bends, we recommend that you rest between repetitions. Simply lie on your belly or back until your breath comes back to ease and your mind and body feel dropped.

The first time you do the practices, we recommend that you sweep through the sequence, doing each pose only once. After that, feel free to extend your practice by repeating poses up to the maximum number of recommended times.

A PLAYFUL PRACTICE

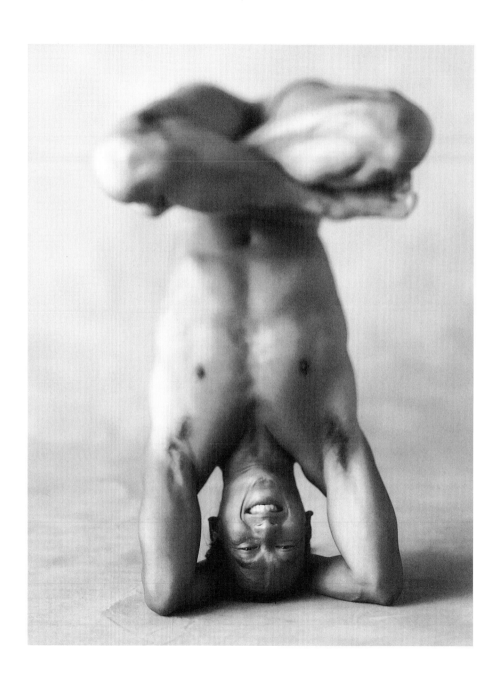

Considering the Practice

*Children pretending to be cormorants
are even more wonderful
than cormorants.*

— ISSA

Playfulness. Yoga doesn't need to be *serious*. You can simply explore and experiment. You can simply be interested and curious. You can simply look at your body and be *in* your body. (And try not to be concerned about what the poses will do for you.)

> *be your body*
> *be your mind*
> *be your breath*

Awareness. As you do your first yoga poses, you start to cultivate your awareness. Let yourself begin the dialogue. Listen and respond. Play. Imagine. Have fun. Assume nothing.

Animal Poses. In yoga you can play at being an animal—feel an animal's or a child's innocent pleasure in the sensations of its splendid body.

Dog Pose

Cat Pose

Lion Pose

Cobra Pose

Happy Baby Pose

Child's Pose

1. Gentle Undulations Lying on Your Back

10 to 15 breaths

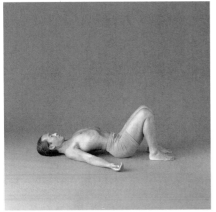

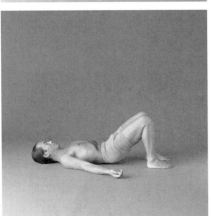

Instructions. On your inhale, drop your sitting bones down toward the ground, lifting the small of your back off the ground. On your exhale, curl your tailbone, pressing the small of your back against the ground.

One Thing. Bring your awareness to your back body and its contact with the ground as you move. *A dog on a summer afternoon rolling on his back on the prickly front lawn, growling with pleasure at finally getting to scratch all those itchy parts.*

2. Mountain Pose, on the Floor

15 to 30 breaths

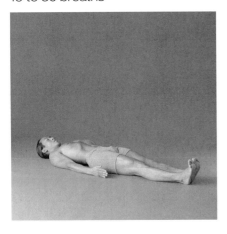

Instructions. Lie on the floor. Reach your legs together, and then extend them strongly through your heels. Spread your toes, wide and alive with sensitivity. Relax your arms down by your sides, with your hands about six inches from your hips. Now observe your body's natural points of contact with the ground, its curves and contours like the silhouette of rolling hills in the twilight.

One Thing. How much can you be connected to the earth, both physically and psychologically? (They say that Mount Tamalpais in California has the form of a sleeping Miwok maiden, and sometimes in the soft light of early evening, we like to gaze at that mountain and daydream about what it must have been like here in those days, before all the building began, before the houses, the bridges, the shopping centers, the freeways . . .).

3. Alternate Knees to Chest
5 to 10 times on each leg

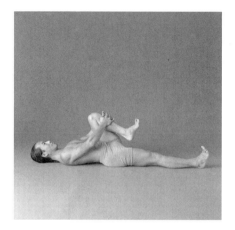

Instructions. Lying on your back, exhale as you use your arms to bring one knee toward your chest. Then inhale as you release your leg back down to the floor. Repeat this with your other leg, exhaling as you bring the knee toward your chest and inhaling as you release it back to the floor. *A pink flamingo drawing one leg into its fluffy, feathery chest.*

One Thing. Observe how the movement of your legs affects your spine. What happens to your lower back? Does the strength of your bottom leg affect the extension of your spine?

4. Random Leg Movements
30 to 60 seconds

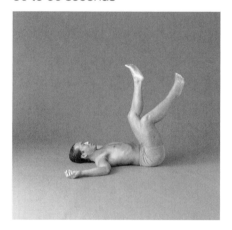

Instructions. Still on your back, move your legs randomly, like an insect stuck on its back trying to right itself, quickly and slowly, with observation.

One Thing. Allow for some spontaneity, and simply listen to your body. What feels pleasant? What hurts? At what points does the deliciousness of moving become discomfort or pain?

5. Happy Baby Pose
15 to 30 breaths

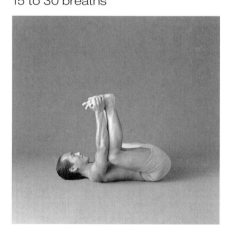

Instructions. Enjoy the feeling of having your spine completely supported as you release your hips. If you cannot easily reach your feet with your hands, modify this pose by using a strap around the arches of your feet.

One Thing. Have you ever watched a six-month-old baby lie on its back and play delightedly with its feet, sometimes even pulling them into its mouth to suck on its toes? Try to return to that body—your baby body—a body with a strong, supple spine and flexible hips.

6. Reclined Twist

15 to 20 breaths per side

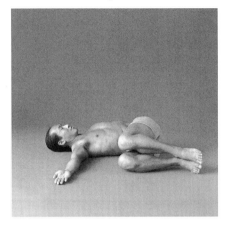

Instructions. Bring both knees together and into your chest, then drop them over to your right. Repeat on the left side.

One Thing. Can you meet the resistance of the twist with release and ease rather than fighting and struggling? *The natural winding of climbing wisteria up and around a trellis.*

7. Reclined Leg Stretch

10 to 20 breaths per side

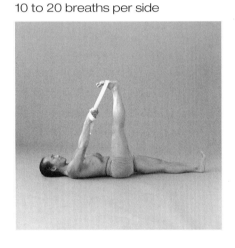

Instructions. With a strap on your right foot, bring your right leg toward your head while extending your left leg vigorously and pressing it down against the ground. Repeat with the left leg.

One Thing. Simply stare at your leg—look at your foot, your shin, your knee, your thigh. Can you see your leg without judgment? Can you just observe your body without criticism? Then play a little with the shape of your foot—twinkle your toes. Remember being a kid and noticing the puppy that someone is walking as you pass by? You are delighted by it and then reach down to pet it.

8. Breathing on Your Belly

10 to 20 breaths

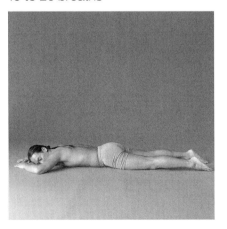

Instructions. Just lie on your belly and breathe, feeling like a beached elephant seal wallowing in the warm sun. (At the halfway point, turn your head to the other side.)

One Thing. Your vital organs are safe now, pressing against the earth and covered by your back. Feel the emotional grounding that comes from being physically grounded. Let your breath come to its natural flow from that connectedness.

9. Modified Cobra
5 to 10 breaths

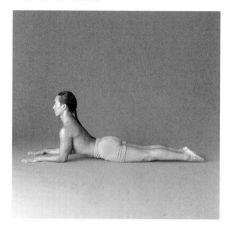

Instructions. Maintaining the grounded quality of the previous pose, elongate your spine. Can you find length and extension of your spine along with relaxation?

One Thing. Let your mind move back into a reptilian consciousness, into a reptilian sinuousness, like a lizard on its belly on hot, dry desert sand.

10. Cat Pose
5 to 10 breaths

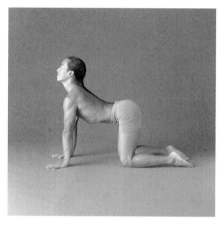

Instructions. On your inhale, drop your pelvis and belly into a soft back bend and then raise your head, like a contented cat. On your exhale, hunch your back and drop your head, like an angry, hissing Halloween cat.

One Thing. Feel the soft, supple muscles, the padded feet, and the prowess of the feline—the energy from the belly of the earth rising and undulating along your spine.

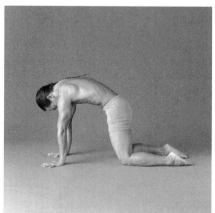

11. Getting Grounded
5 to 10 times per hand

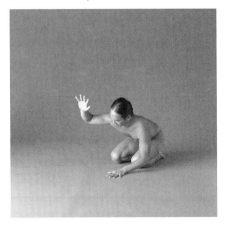

Instructions. Sitting on your heels, lean forward and slap your relaxed hands repeatedly on the ground, like an orangutan pounding on the jungle floor. Can you touch the floor evenly throughout both your hands, connecting your whole body to the earth *through* your hands?

One Thing. Wake up your hands (and your body) through the sting of a slap.

12. Child's Pose
15 to 30 breaths

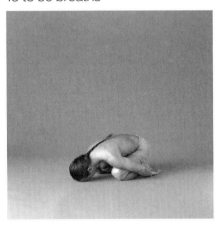

Instructions. With your knees slightly apart and big toes together, bring your sitting bones toward your heels so your spine releases over your legs like an embryo in the womb. If your contact with the floor is uncomfortable, do the pose on a folded blanket.

One Thing. Play at hiding. Remember how small children play peek-a-boo? How they think that if they can't see you—if they are hiding their eyes behind their hands—you can't see them?

13. Lion Pose
3 to 5 roars

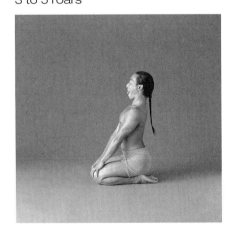

Instructions. Stick your tongue out toward your chin, as far as it can go. Cross your eyes to stare at the tip of your nose. On your exhale, roar like a lion, letting the sound come from the very depths of your intestines.

One Thing. Feel the depth of your belly—the lion's roar resounding through your entire body.

14. Downward-Facing Dog
10 to 25 breaths

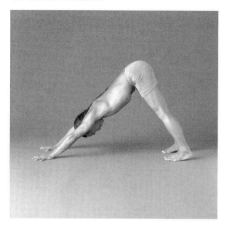

Instructions. Shift your weight from one hand to the other and from one foot to the other, and search for a place where your hands and feet are evenly grounded. Then alternate between just feeling and observing the pose and continuing to search for evenness.

One Thing. Bring a lightness to this pose, a feeling of suspension, the way a sudden cool breeze brings you relief as you're working in the garden on a hot sweaty day.

15. Standing Forward Bend, with Bent Legs
10 to 15 breaths

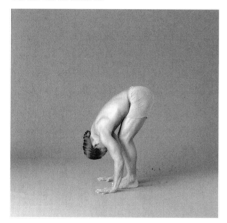

Instructions. From Downward-Facing Dog, prowl forward into Standing Forward Bend, with bent legs.

One Thing. Bring your awareness to the touch of the soles of your feet sensuously contacting the ground. *Sitting on the end of a dock, dangling your feet in a cool summer lake.*

16. Standing Forward Bend, with Straight Legs

10 to 15 breaths

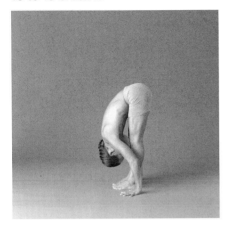

Instructions. Still in Standing Forward Bend, slowly straighten your legs.

One Thing. Let your head hang easily and comfortably, like a gazelle bending to graze contentedly on wild grasses.

17. Tree Pose

7 to 15 breaths per side

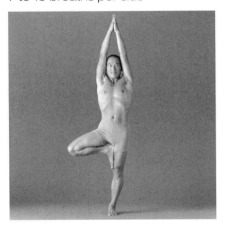

Instructions. From a basic standing position, bring one foot high into the groin of your other leg. When you are ready, reach your arms above your head.

One Thing. Be a tree swaying in the wind—and maybe falling (it's good to fall). Feel the movement, your weight shifting, your body moving back and forth. Play with falling to all sides—left, right, backward and forward.

18. Mountain Pose

15 to 30 breaths

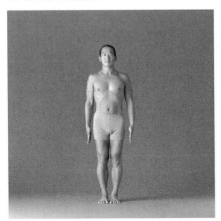

Instructions. Stand with your legs together and your feet spread open, as tenacious as an eagle's talons. Let your waist grow long, and lift and open your chest.

One Thing. Bring yourself home now—home to the mountain, home to your body—with a sense of ease and contentment. Retain the broad vision of the mountain, looking out over all creation.

19. Relaxation Pose

5 to 10 minutes

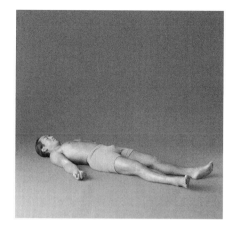

Instructions. Lie on your back, creating as much symmetry as possible between the right and left sides of your body. Then, with your eyes closed, wiggle around until you feel very comfortable and the skin of your back is resting easily on the ground.

One Thing. Remember when you were a child and you would pretend to be asleep because you knew your parents would *carry* you to bed if they thought you were sleeping (and make you *walk* if they thought you were awake)? And when your parents lifted you up (maybe from the car on the way home from your grandma's or from their bed after story time was finished), you would let yourself go totally limp, feeling completely relaxed, safe and secure in the warmth of their embrace? And maybe your parents knew that you were only pretending to be asleep—and you knew that they knew—but you both kept on pretending because it was such a sweet, delicious moment?

In Relaxation Pose, allow yourself to drop into that feeling.

20. Sitting Meditation

5 minutes or intuition

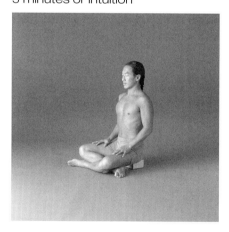

Sitting. Sit in a simple crossed-legged position on a block with your hands on your thighs. Play with your sitting posture until you find a position that is new—not your habitual posture—but that is also comfortable enough for you to maintain for an extended period of time.

One Thing. For this first time, try to sit for five minutes and just enjoy your monkey mind. Observe your wandering, leaping mind. Your curious, playful mind. Notice and enjoy the daydreams, the boundless movement of your mind.

Reconsidering the Practice

Playing is a way to gain different perspectives. So as you move through your day, try on new ways of moving, of breathing, and of thinking, as you would put on costumes from a dress-up trunk.

Use different gestures and bigger movements. Be more animated. Express more with your hands. And when you are walking, swing your arms more, sway your hips more.

Be playful with your breath. Take a deep breath every so often. Try holding your breath as long as you can. Or try to breathe as quietly and minimally as possible, as if you were hiding from lions.

In conversations, listen deeply to the other person instead of arguing your own point of view (you already know what *you* think), or take someone else's point of view just to play with some new ideas.

And when you practice yoga, let your mind take different shapes just as your body does. Can you play with your body-mind, with the way you are used to thinking about your body? If you think you are tight, be flexible. If you think you are weak, be strong. If you think you are afraid, be courageous. Start by pretending.

How do small children play? Wholeheartedly. From the playground you can hear it all: their shrieks of laughter, their shouts of anger, their tears of sadness. So why not play that way, too? Why not feel everything wholeheartedly?

GETTING LOST TOGETHER

Where I was, where I am, wherever I go—I always picture myself on a great, curving, three-dimensional map, and, on a crisp fall evening with a clear, round moon, where would I be without my place here at the eastern edge of the San Francisco Bay, just across from Mount Tamalpais, that stern, implacable presence—but once when I was a child, I followed another girl and let her take me so far into the foothills that we got lost—in a canyon in West Los Angeles (the sharp, earthy smell of sage—the crumbly granite, the dry dusty earth—the tall, proud spikes of yucca, the scrubby sumac, the sticky orange monkey flowers—the howling of a coyote, the glimpse of a deer crashing through the brush, the tiny gray lizards scooting across the jagged outcroppings)—"Come on," she told me, "there will be bunnies and policemen to take care of us," and so I went with her, enchanted (the sky dazzling blue and the clouds spun sugar, the dusty earth shimmering gold, and the milky quartz moonstones gleaming), and walked on and on behind her, wordlessly, dazed and dreamy, and lost all track of our turnings, until she said, "Oh, no!" and "I think we're lost" and "This doesn't look right and I don't know where we are," and threw herself down on the dirt, helplessly sobbing, and with that my mind was suddenly cleared—I didn't even mention the policemen—and when she would not get up, I left her on that hillside and followed a path down, down, wherever it went down, and came back with a woman I had found to rescue her, and there she was, still there, still crying, and so we took her home—and for many years I thought that our getting lost together meant something about the two of us, my friend and me, maybe that she was fantasy and I was reality or maybe that she was art and I was dry fact, but now I don't think so anymore, now I think that I loved her and that what happened was only that—what happened.

—NINA ZOLOTOW

Playful Practice Summary

1. Gentle Undulations, Lying on Your Back
10 to 15 breaths

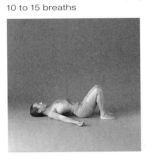

2. Mountain Pose, on the Floor
15 to 30 breaths

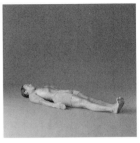

3. Alternate Knees to Chest
5 to 10 times on each leg

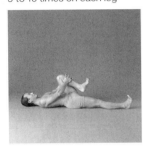

4. Random Leg Movements
30 to 60 seconds

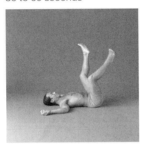

5. Happy Baby Pose
15 to 30 breaths

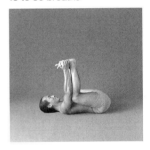

6. Reclined Twist
15 to 20 breaths per side

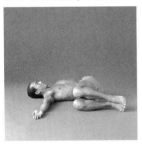

7. Reclined Leg Stretch
10 to 20 breaths per side

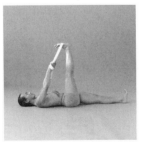

8. Breathing on Your Belly
10 to 20 breaths

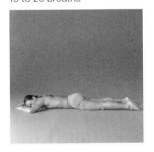

9. Modified Cobra
5 to 10 breaths

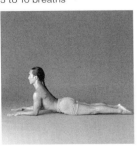

10. Cat Pose
5 to 10 breaths

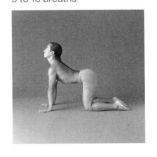
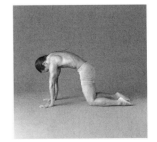

11. Getting Grounded
5 to 10 times per hand

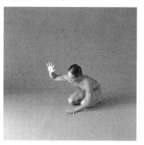

12. Child's Pose
15 to 30 breaths

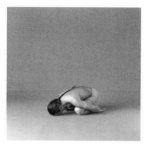

13. Lion Pose
3 to 5 roars

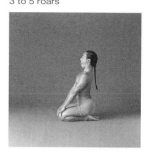

14. Downward-Facing Dog
10 to 25 breaths

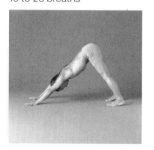

15. Standing Forward Bend, with Bent Legs
10 to 15 breaths

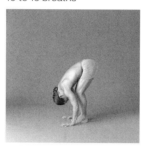

16. Standing Forward Bend, with Straight Legs
10 to 15 breaths

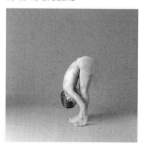

17. Tree Pose
7 to 15 breaths per side

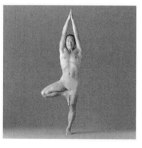

18. Mountain Pose
15 to 30 breaths

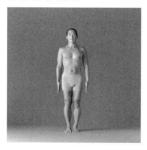

19. Relaxation Pose
5 to 10 minutes

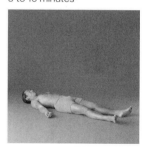

20. Sitting Meditation
5 minutes or intuition

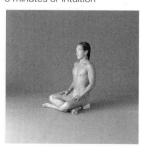

No Right Conversations

NINA   When you started asking me to talk about my yoga practice, it was really difficult for me. I have never talked about my practice to anyone before. And I've never practiced with anyone before. As a matter of fact, I've always been sort of secretive about it because . . . well, I was afraid I wasn't doing it *right.*

ROD   This might be the number one dilemma for people practicing at home: am I doing things right? You weren't with me at my workshop in Virginia, Nina, but I know I told you this story. I kept on asking people there, "Where is your breath?" And they kept on telling me where they *wanted* it to be. And I kept on saying, "No, that's not what I'm asking. I'm asking just where *is* it?" And there was so much resistance to that, to just saying where it *was.* And finally, one woman got all shaken up—one of the more advanced practitioners, actually—and she said, "I just want to know where you *want* us to breathe because I just want to do it right!"

     And I was really glad that came up because I find that so many people are doing this in their yoga practice and probably in every aspect of their lives—they're always trying to do their life right. And somewhere in their minds, they've got an idea of how to do it right, and they think they need to stay on that line, that razor's edge.

     Let's address this first in the yoga practice itself. Again, the postures are a conversation. They're a dialogue, so it's not like someone's *right* in the dialogue. It's more like you're having a conversation, for instance, with center, as in A Falling Practice in this book. Of course, you're never in the exact center. There is no exact center. It's a matter of feeling how the body gets more and more aligned, and then it gets out of that alignment, and then you bring it back into that alignment. And then you refine it even more into the subtle level of where the infinite center is, and then again you fall out and you fall back in, and you fall back out in different ways and to different extents. And so it's not about getting it right, it's about listening and responding.

NINA   What about the beginner who's worried that he somehow doesn't have enough information about the poses just from looking at the pictures in this book and reading the short descriptions that go along with them? And what about the person who is concerned that he might hurt himself or create some problems because he doesn't know how to do it "right"?

ROD   I think there is a concern about doing it right because people are a bit worried about getting hurt, and they think that if they don't do the pose properly they will get hurt. You know, we *do* live in a physical universe where there seem to be certain principles or laws of physics, like gravity. You drop something; it falls to the earth. And in some ways, the alignment of our human body has some principles that can guide you in your dialogue with the posture. So hopefully in this book we present enough guidelines and signposts to give you an orientation that is healthy for the human body. But even while we are giving you this orientation, it's still about you exploring your body—this is where these concepts come alive. Of course, the pictures will help you, but sometimes, you know, we do the external shape but we're not really having the internal dialogue. So I'm trying to, in this book, help guide people into having a dialogue as well as giving them the guidelines.

NINA   What if something feels really awful? What if a person starts trying to do a pose that's in the book and it just feels really miserable or even excruciating?

ROD   A lot of times people think that unless a pose hurts, it's not doing any good—no pain, no gain. But this is a very Western idea. In fact, in yoga, one of the principles is to do the poses with ease. And when you do the poses with ease—in other words, when you modify the pose or come out of the pose until it's somewhat easy for you (not just going for what the picture looks like or what someone has told you to do)—there's actually more capability of observing the pose and making more subtle adjustments and starting to come to some understanding instead of just fighting the pose or pushing the pose. So if something feels really horrible, I would say probably come out of the pose enough so that you can have a sense of enjoyment and relief in the pose.

Now there are some poses in which you have to struggle—I mean in which you have to build muscle or flexibility or learn about relaxation. And I do encourage you to go into some of the poses that are difficult for you. But go into them with a sense of exploration and a sense of curiosity, not for a sense of achievement or pushing.

NINA   So there is some relationship between listening to your body enough while you are doing a difficult pose—let's say, the back bend called Bow Pose— and going slowly enough so you know when to back off.

ROD   Yes. In this book we've picked beginning postures that are accessible to most people, but at the same time there are poses that are quite challenging. So you might get into the pose and you might feel a lot of strain in one area of your body. If that's happening while you're practicing, you should try to distribute the opening more evenly throughout the body. So when you're doing a back bend like a Bow Pose, if your lower back is getting most of the stress, see if you can let your lower back *not* bend as much, but maybe bend more in the hips or the upper chest. Usually when there's a heavy pain or heavy sensation in one area of the body, it means there's another part of your body that you're not working. So you want to take that pain and try to distribute the work evenly throughout the posture till it feels more equalized, not localized.

NINA   You've been talking in class lately about how the ego makes people want to try to do the pose deeper, if you know what I mean.

ROD   Let me say something about *deeper* first. To me, when a pose is deeper, it doesn't mean that you're stretching more intensely—for example, if you're forward bending, that your head is closer to your shins. Deeper to me is when there's more synchronicity between the breath, the body, and the mind. What we're trying to do in yoga is to create a union, and so to deepen a yoga pose is to actually increase the union of the pose, not necessarily put your leg around your head.

NINA   Yes, but I remember hearing a woman who had been just once to one of your classes say, "Oh my God, I went to the beginning class and I was in the back row and there were all these people in the front row wearing these perfect little outfits and they all put their legs right behind their heads." She felt completely intimidated and discouraged by that. So I think people feel like that's what they need to achieve in order to really be doing "yoga."

ROD   Well, I guess we have to face reality in the sense that a lot of us, you know, compare ourselves with other people in class. We start comparing ourselves and saying, "Oh, they can do this and I can't do that, and I wish I could do that, and if I push really hard maybe I can do that." But you have to realize that in some ways your tightness or your difficulty is your blessing, because when you come against your boundaries, you really have to look at yourself. And that's an important aspect of yoga, not just on a physical level of putting your legs and arms in ways that you've seen other people do. It's more about coming against your boundaries, and breathing and centering yourself when you come up against your boundaries. So I always say that a tight person has the advantage because they don't have to look as bizarre as they come up against their boundaries. The person who's in the front row and has their leg behind their head, you know, they're also coming up against their boundary—their boundary just tends to be in a different place, but it's still a place that they have to look at and figure out. Their boundary might be their flexibility—they might be overflexible. It's important to have stability, too, and a lot of flexible people are not as stable and not as oriented in their bodies and might lack a sense of center. So they might have completely different difficulties that arise from what you see as their gifts.

    I have to explain this a lot to people who think that mastering yoga means to be extremely flexible—I have to explain that it's a combination of flexibility and strength and relaxation. We're trying to balance the body, not trying to stretch it more and more and more. The reason why the poses get more difficult is that you do get to some mastery, and so you go on and move into a more difficult pose, again to elicit your boundary, to keep on coming against the boundary, not necessarily to go through it.

    Are you competitive in yoga class?

NINA   Yes, sometimes. But sometimes I'm not. I think most of the time when I'm in the class I'm not really looking at other people and I'm trying to work on my own, being competitive with myself mainly.

ROD   Are there any poses that you feel like you've mastered?

NINA   No.

ROD   Does the word *mastery* even come into your mind when you're doing the practice?

NINA   No, because I feel that even with the simplest poses I'm still working on things. It is interesting for me, as I take both your beginning class and your advanced class, and in a way I find the beginning class more difficult, more demanding. I think this is because you have us move through more poses more quickly in the advanced class, so sometimes there are parts of it that are more like a workout, while the beginning class requires more mindfulness because it is slower and requires more concentration on subtle movements of the body.

ROD   I think that has something to do with doing things right. See, some people in interviews and so forth have said to me, "Oh, you know, you're seen as a master yogi and—"

NINA   They use that word, *master?*

ROD   Yes, they call me a "yoga master," and I sort of laugh under my breath because I think, what have I mastered? I don't even understand that concept. I don't feel like I've mastered anything, or I don't feel like I'm even trying to master anything—I don't even know what that means. It's just an ongoing exploration. I might see someone do a pose that I haven't done before or do it in a different way than I've done it, and I think, oh, that's really interesting, I want to explore that. Let's say that you can do a posture—like you, for instance, have done Downward-Facing Dog a thousand times, so it might seem to an outsider like you've "mastered it"—and there is a certain level of knowledge and competence—however, the more you practice it, the more you sense its infinite nuances. So it's endless, really. It's an endless journey of your curiosity.

So I think you're beginning to see that there is not even a question of "doing it right" anymore. It's funny that you didn't even want to tell me—or share with anyone—how you practice at home, because you might have the possibility of, oh, shoot, I'm doing it wrong. But in some sense if you just practice at home, you start realizing, now wait, there's not really any "wrong" here. I'm just in these poses, and I'm playing with them and discovering more things about them, and they're talking to me, I'm talking to them, and all of a sudden your practice is over and it's not about trying to do something right. It's like saying, oh, "You and I are going to have a talk, and we're going to try to have a *right* conversation." Wouldn't that be sort of a strange thing, to label it as a *right conversation?*

NINA   Well, yes, but there are some conversations that are better than others—

ROD   Yes, but even though we might say, oh, "We had a good conversation," that doesn't mean we had a *right* conversation.

NINA   Yes. Well, one of the things that I was embarrassed about is that during my home practice, I listen to music while I practice, so—

ROD   That's definitely wrong!

NINA   [laughs]

ROD   We don't use music in class, so you felt like you were—?

NINA   Cheating.

ROD   Cheating. For what reason?

NINA   Because it made me want to practice more. And it made me enjoy my practice more to have music. So—

ROD   That's completely permitted, you know—to enjoy yourself while doing yoga—

NINA   So lately I decided that I would—because of our talks probably—get over it, and I started dancing while I was doing yoga, too, just dancing around to the music.

ROD   Sounds like you're doing the practice right!

NINA   [laughs]

ROD   You know, when you spend some time with yourself, listening to your body, you'll begin to feel that there are certain things coming *out* from your body, like wisdom, memories, feelings, and thoughts. And if you respond to those internal risings, then when you practice, you might spontaneously take different yoga shapes. So in some sense, doing yoga is allowing your body to respond to all that, letting your body respond to thoughts, letting your body respond to music, letting your body respond to emotions, so it really becomes physical configurations of *internal* motions.

        And when you start getting more familiar with the poses, you start realizing, oh, well, I feel this way and so I'm going to do these poses. It's just an intuitive thing, like, oh, I feel a little depressed and I think I want to elicit some energy in my body, so I'm going to do some back bends. Or, I'm feeling confused and ungrounded, so maybe I should do some standing poses. Or, God, my mind is wild today—it's racing around—so maybe I should do a practice of Sun Salutations and intersperse it with standing poses and back bends, and maybe my mind will drop into the present moment. So the *appropriate* practice is really just a matter of listening and beginning to understand the postures that deal with your current state of being.

NINA   But I have to say that even knowing all of this, it is still really hard to let go of the need to try to do things right. Even while I'm by myself at home, I might fail to do some new pose that I'm working on—like a balance pose— or I might fall down in a pose I think I should be able to do, and I feel a sudden rush of shame. I'm all by myself and I feel this terrible shame that I can't do the pose right.

ROD   So the conversation is just that. You feel ashamed, and that's the feeling that you're listening to and responding to. It's not that you need to get rid of that feeling or any other feeling. Can we accept all that it means to be human?

A FALLING PRACTICE

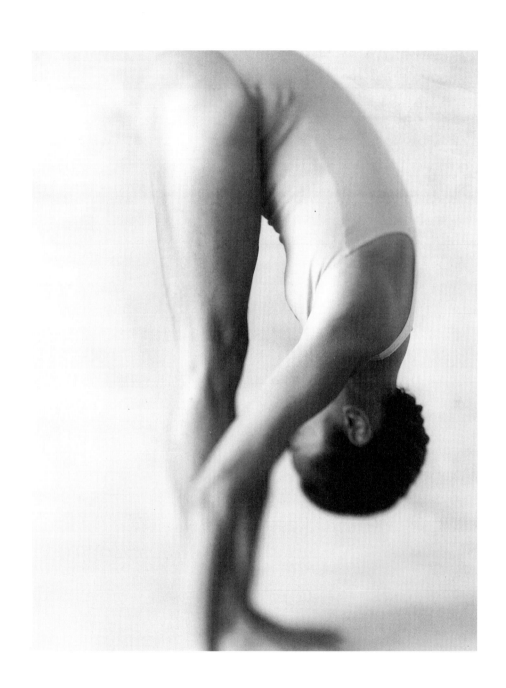

Considering the Practice

I will tell you what he told me
in the years just after the war
as we then called
the second world war

don't lose your arrogance yet he said
you can do that when you're older
lose it too soon and you may
merely replace it with vanity

just one time he suggested
changing the usual order
of the same words in a line of verse
why point out a thing twice

he suggested I pray to the Muse
get down on my knees and pray
right there in the corner and he
said he meant it literally

it was in the days before the beard
and the drink but he was deep
in tides of his own through which he sailed
chin sideways and head tilted like a tacking sloop

he was far older than the dates allowed for
much older than I was he was in his thirties
he snapped down his nose with an accent
I think he had affected in England

as for publishing he advised me
to paper my wall with rejection slips
his lips and the bones of his long fingers trembled
with vehemence of his view about poetry

he said the great presence
that permitted everything and transmuted it
in poetry was passion
passion was genius and he praised movement and
    invention

I had hardly begun to read
I asked how can you ever be sure
that what you write is really
any good at all and he said you can't

you can't you can never be sure
you die without knowing
whether anything you wrote was any good
if you have to be sure don't write

—W. S. MERWIN

Falling. Falling is what is always happening. To *hold* a yoga pose is not possible; it's a sensuous dance, moment by moment. And rigidity is simply the illusion that we can create a world in which we're not falling.

Can you mindfully practice falling? Falling away from your habits, falling out of your habits? Can you play with center? Question center? Use falling as a way to question what you think of as center?

Centering. Center is not a place but a dialogue. Your dialogue with the floor and sometimes with the wall. The dialogue between your mind and your body. A playful dialogue. A relaxed dialogue. A curious dialogue.

Can you observe and respond? Pose and repose? Can you *be* in the pose instead of *doing* the pose? Can you let yourself shimmer in the center?

Balance. Balance is your ability to fall and then retrieve yourself. As you fall out of center and then into it and then out of it—again and again—you may begin to lose your old sense of orientation. And to feel fear. Fear of what? Of change? Of not knowing? Of losing control?

These poses allow you to play with falling and centering, centering and falling:

Mountain Pose

Tree Pose

Triangle Pose

Half-Moon Pose

1. Relaxation Pose

1 to 5 minutes

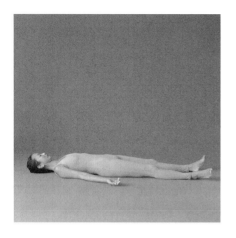

Instructions. Feel your natural curves against the ground. Observe what touches the ground (head, shoulder blades, buttocks, legs, heels?) and what is slightly off the ground (lower back, neck, tailbone?). Intentionally shift your body to create as much broadness, length, symmetry, and ease as possible. Once your back body feels supported, let your front body fall into it like a pillow to which you surrender the weight of your head.

Then, as you exhale, feel the weight of your entire body fall. Can you keep falling and falling until every strand of tension has unraveled? Ask yourself: what am I, the holding or the falling?

One Thing. Let your breath flow along the riverbed of your body, and your mind fall into your breath as it flows.

2. Mountain Pose, Against the Wall

15 to 25 breaths

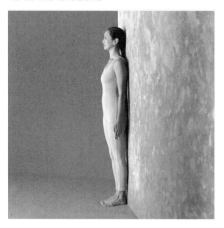

Instructions. Touch the back of your head, your shoulder blades, the section of the spine between your shoulder blades, and your buttocks to the wall. Now observe what is slightly off the wall (lower back, neck, tailbone, legs, heels?). Try pressing different parts of your body into the wall—what feels most balanced?

Play with the evenness of your weight between your right and left foot. Then fall into your contact with the wall and lengthen up the wall. Use the wall as a reference in your exploration of center. *Shimmer in the center of your balance.*

One Thing. Close your eyes and feel your breath undulate along the natural curves of your spine, of your back body, against the wall.

3. Mountain Pose,
Away from the Wall
15 to 25 breaths

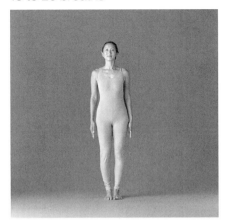

Instructions. As you stand, fall forward, backward, left, and right. Where do you feel the weight on your feet? Do you know where your habit is, where you usually stand? On your left foot? On your right foot? On the outside of your feet? On the inside of your feet? On your heels? On your toes?

Practice making the pose strong without making it rigid. Let your muscles move you toward center as you retain the sense of falling. Lift and open your heart with suppleness, feeling your breath sway you as a wind moves a branch.

One Thing. Let yourself fall and recover, fall and recover, fall and recover, retrieving your balance, refining your balance, falling into the center of your balance.

4. Standing Forward Bend
10 to 15 breaths

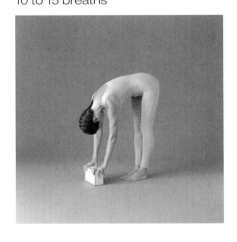

Instructions. Let your torso, your head, and your arms fall completely downward, balanced by the grounding of your legs. Re-find your center somewhere between the weight of your body and the strength of your legs. Do you feel that your orientation has shifted dramatically—upside down and inward?

Not only is this an inversion (you are upside down), but the roles of your front body and back body are reversed. The back body, which normally supports the openness of the front body, is now opened and supported by the front body. In this reversal of your typical orientation, can you surrender and fall into these sensations?

One Thing. As you fall into this new orientation, let the movement of your breath bring awareness to a forsaken part of your body.

5. Downward-Facing Dog
15 to 30 breaths

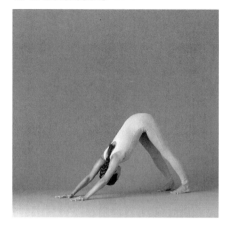

Instructions. Before you extend the pose, feel the weight of your body drop into your hands and your feet. With this sense of falling, actively reach your hands into the ground in one direction and pull your thighs back in the opposite direction. Now feel the weight of your pelvis falling into your feet, and, from this grounding, gather the energy through the conduits of your legs back up into your pelvis. Feel the muscles of your arms and legs center around their bones, and harness the energy of your extremities into the center of your spine.

One Thing. Feel your weight falling evenly onto each foot, onto each hand, onto every finger. *The pinnacle of a pyramid rising from the solid foundation of four sides.*

6. Hero Pose
15 to 30 breaths

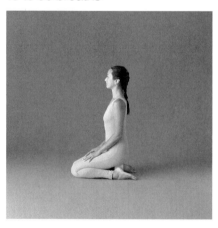

Instructions. Feel the front of your shins being forced downward, your thighbones falling into your hamstrings and your hamstrings falling into the earth. Spill your pelvis slightly forward, initiating the natural curves of your spine. Can you remember the natural curves of your spine in Relaxation Pose and in Mountain Pose?

Your legs are like the compacted root ball of an unplanted tree. But from that density, there is a strong weightedness toward the center of the earth. This falling into the pose—a relaxation into the pose—can sustain circulation even as your legs fold and press together so densely.

One Thing. Find your balance through the equanimity of the surrender of both of your thighs, of their falling.

7. Tree Pose

10 to 15 breaths per side
Repetitions: 1 to 2 times on each
side (right and left, then right
and left again)

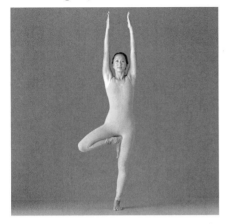

Instructions. The aliveness and the growing of Tree Pose comes from your ability to allow the juxtaposition of your legs falling into the center of the earth while your torso and arms reach skyward. Play with intentionally falling out of this pose (forward, backward, right, and left). Maybe even with your eyes closed. Maybe even backward with your eyes closed.

Are you really afraid of falling, or have you been taught to be afraid of falling? Is your idea of success in this pose staying up on one leg? Where are you clutching, grabbing, and clenching? Where do you carry your habitual tension in the face of falling? Can you just continue to play with the nebulous center?

One Thing. Be like a child first learning to walk, willing to try over and over again, relaxed and innocent in the face of falling.

8. Triangle Pose

10 to 15 breaths per side
Repetitions: 1 to 2 times on each
side (right and left, then right and
left again)

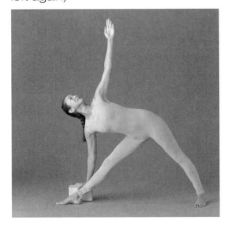

Instructions. Most people feel fairly stable in this pose, but this stability often comes from being contracted toward the front body. So bring your head behind your heart and your heart in the same plane as your pelvis. Then play with falling back slightly, searching for a new center. Balance the amount of weight on your right and left feet, and feel the connection between the center of each leg and the center of your spine.

Search for an alignment where your torso is in the same plane as your legs. And try to balance your top arm right over the foundation of your bottom arm. Can you feel the vulnerability of your heart?

One Thing. The architecture of the triangle is strong and steady, but continue to feel the dialogue of center and falling.

9. Half-Moon Pose

5 to 10 breaths on each side
Repetitions: 1 to 2 times on each
side (right and left, then right
and left again)

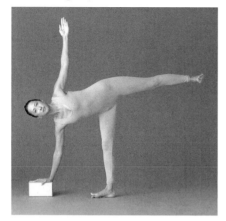

Instructions. Keep your bottom leg turned out, your top leg strong, and your head, chest, and buttocks lined up with the heel of your raised leg.

Fear becomes dominant in this pose, which makes you tend to turn your standing leg in, let your body fall forward of center, and collapse your raised leg. The natural tendency of your body is to take a shape that will ensure that you fall on your butt if you fall backward. But this is a fearful balance, not an open balance.

Can you let go of the fear caging your heart—the fear of falling backward, the fear of falling into the unseen, the fear of falling into the unknown?

One Thing. Can you be with the fear in the center of your falling? Then you find your ease. Then you soar.

10. Relaxation Pose

5 to 10 minutes

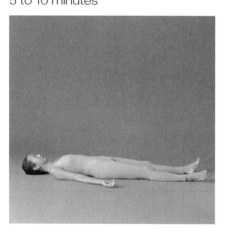

Instructions. Let your legs fall first. Then your arms. Then your belly. Then your torso. Then your head. Feel the imprint of your entire body sinking deeper into soft earth. Even though you are on the ground, you can begin to feel like you are floating between the earth and the sky. Let go of your familiar physical identity. Fall completely. When you are falling, what are you surrendering?

One Thing. You can fall now without retrieving yourself, so keep falling and falling and falling. Can you calculate the space inside yourself—the night sky inside your mind? Can you sense the depth of the ocean in your breath? The belly rising and falling? And can you understand the richness of the earth by knowing your legs, your arms, your torso, your neck, your head. . .?

11. Sitting Meditation

5 minutes or intuition

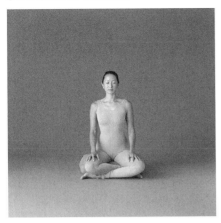

Sitting. Sit in a simple crossed-legged position, on a prop that is high enough so your pelvis and spine can fall in any direction and feel like they are floating in the center. Waver in and out of the natural curves of your spine, allowing your spine to wander and then readjust itself—feeling the weight of your head over your torso and the weight of your torso over your sitting bones as your legs fall into the earth.

Meditating. Let the center of your meditation be your breath—allow yourself to fall into thoughts and then bring yourself back to your breath (when your thoughts travel freely, they will come home).

Reconsidering the Practice

When you feel that your life is out of balance, can you still search for center—fall in and out of it and then back in again?

> *Wander*
> *Waver*
> *Glisten*
> *Glimmer*
> *Dazzle*
> *Shimmer*

Can you fall out of your habits and recenter in new places? If you go the same way to work, try a different way—take the "long cut" for a change. If you are always late, show up fifteen minutes early. If you always talk, shut up and listen. If you always listen, speak up. Because falling can be synonymous with taking a chance or with allowing yourself to be completely spontaneous.

And what are some of your physical habits? When you are talking, do you cross your arms in front of your heart? Or hold your wrists behind your back? Or put your hands in your pockets? Try letting your arms dangle by your sides and feel the uneasiness that arises. The ability to deal with this uneasiness is an important aspect of breaking your habits and recentering. Besides, what's so scary about going to a physical place that's unknown—isn't that happening all the time?

What are the physical centers of your life (*your body, your bed, your kitchen, the earth you plow each spring, the flowering dogwood tree you planted twenty years ago, the ocean waves crashing against the rocky coast of Maine, the view of Mount Tamalpais from your second-story window*)?

What are the emotional centers of your life (*your lover, your children, your friends, your faith, your job, your garden, your art, your writing, your running, your dancing, your solitude*)?

What are the philosophical centers of your life (*your politics, your ethics, your religion, your poetry, your love, your convictions, your doubts*)?

Can you allow yourself to fall out of these physical, emotional, and philosophical centers? Because ultimately, holding on to what is and continuing with your habitual patterns may *feel* secure, but what are you securing? Maybe only rigidity, boredom, depression, stagnation, or despair. But if you consciously acknowledge that every unfolding moment is a movement into the unknown and that you need a new set of responses to dance in its rhythm, you will be able to savor the passing of all the seasons—spring, summer, fall, and winter—in all their peculiar and fleeting glories.

R U THE ONE?

Attractive, petite, 30-something SWF seeks 30-something, nonsmoking SM, any race, to meet me over café au lait served in white French coffee bowls so we can sit under a grape arbor and discuss books, films, our childhoods, and our previous relationships, and feel that sudden, surprising connection that seems to come only once in a lifetime, where the talk flows between us as if we have known each other since birth and what we share in common is so much more important than our differences, which will lead to further dates (walking on the sand at Stinson Beach, lunch at Tra Vigne in the wine country, gazing out at the view of the bay and Mount Tamalpais from the Berkeley rose garden) and long conversations at night in bed, until my feelings for u grow so intense that I will begin to feel scared and, over falafel at a Mediterranean restaurant, I will confess that fear to u—I don't know whether or not I can trust u, I will say—and u will take my hand and make promises to me (love, trust, believe me, I won't, really, yes, absolutely?); but only a few days later, u will phone and say that u have changed your mind, that u want to call it off, that after all u aren't yet ready for a committed LTR, and even though I am heartbroken and confused (why will u have said all that if u didn't really mean it?), and think of u first thing upon waking every morning, I will make a point of going again to all the places we will have gone together—the restaurants, the parks, the viewpoints where we will have looked out and had long talks—because I will be determined not to let my painful memories of u deprive me of anything, although there will be one place I will not be able to summon up enough courage even to enter for years—the Mediterranean restaurant—since the last time we will have been there will be when u made all those promises to me, promises the exact words of which I will not be able to remember as time passes, though I will remember well enough that the very thought of falafel, something I will have once loved, makes me feel sick to my stomach, until one day, I will finally enter the place with a friend from work, will order falafel, peel back the silver wrapping, and begin to eat, slowly and carefully, and it will be fine.

—NINA ZOLOTOW

Falling Practice Summary

1. Relaxation Pose
1 to 5 minutes

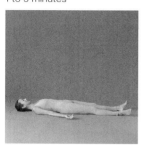

2. Mountain Pose, Against the Wall
15 to 25 breaths

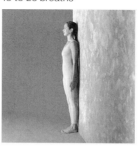

3. Mountain Pose, Away from the Wall
15 to 25 breaths

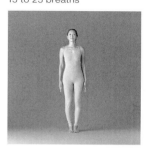

4. Standing Forward Bend
10 to 15 breaths

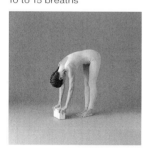

5. Downward-Facing Dog
15 to 30 breaths

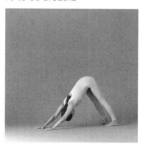

6. Hero Pose
15 to 30 breaths

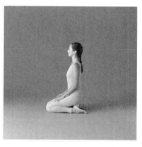

7. Tree Pose
10 to 15 breaths per side, 1 to 2 times

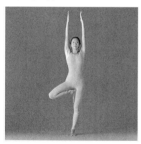

8. Triangle Pose
10 to 15 breaths per side, 1 to 2 times

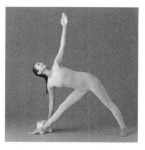

9. Half-Moon Pose
5 to 10 breaths on each side, 1 to 2 times

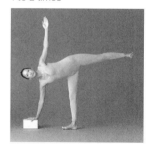

10. Relaxation Pose
5 to 10 minutes

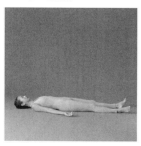

11. Sitting Meditation
5 minutes or intuition

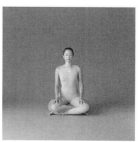

Coconut Ice Cream

ROD This summer I'm planning to go to Bali with my family and I'm planning to go to China with my son. I'm looking forward to it and I'm excited about it, but what if, right before we get on the plane, I just don't feel like going because some internal thing says, "God, I just don't want to go"? The thing is, because I've planned everything, that's what I'm going to get. But it's so great to go out sometimes, not knowing what's going to happen, and respond not to what you expected to see but to the environment as it is. It's like when I see some people go to Europe and they've already read everything in the tour book that they're going to see, so they just end up going to those places. "I'm going to go see the Eiffel Tower, the Louvre . . ." and that's my Paris trip—that's Paris. Why not just wander—at least have a couple of days when you just wander around on the street, when you don't know where you're going to eat, when you don't even know what time you're going to get up or go to sleep?

NINA Well, that's the idea behind my search for coconut ice cream when I go to Hawaii. Because there's so much there. . . . I could read the guidebooks and decide that I need to see this and that, and I could rush around. So it's a joke with me, but it's symbolic. I always say, I don't care what I do as long as I get coconut ice cream at some point.

ROD So you allow the rest of the trip to be free.

NINA   Yes, exactly. And that means if I'm with someone who feels they need to see this or do that, they can do whatever they want and that's fine with me. Obviously, if I came to Hawaii and I didn't eat coconut ice cream—

ROD   —it might not kill your life. So that's sort of the theme of this book, really. All through this book, we have "one thing." And the theme is "one thing" not in the sense of that's all you're going to find, but in fact, it's about not having such a big agenda, so you can allow yourself to see what is arising. But having at least one thing, though, gives you an orientation from which other things can arise. So if I'm deciding in one practice to just look at my feet, well, in a practice of looking just at my feet and feeling just with my feet and playing just with my feet, I start realizing, oh my gosh, that just one thing with my feet is affecting my knees. And that just one thing with my feet is actually affecting my mind and the way I stand, my posture. But if you have too much of an agenda, in some sense you don't see anything. You end up just running around fulfilling your agenda, and you are never even present.

And that's why we've created the Falling Practice, to help people realize that when you do yoga it's important to trust your intuition instead of always having an agenda, a set sequence, in which you're going to just paint by the numbers. It might be good just to listen or play and feel what arises. This might seem advanced, and confusing at first, and even, possibly, disturbing, but these are all aspects that are associated with not knowing. If you go into the practice realizing that you don't know, just as you might walk around a city that you're not familiar with, then you're prepared for being lost. You don't get frustrated about not knowing because you don't expect yourself to know. This allows you to use curiosity and exploration as the foundation for your movement and action.

Falling from the present moment into the next moment. Falling from the observation of what is into the unknown.

So that's what we're trying to say in this book. We don't have to know what yoga is. We just fall into it.

A GROUNDING PRACTICE

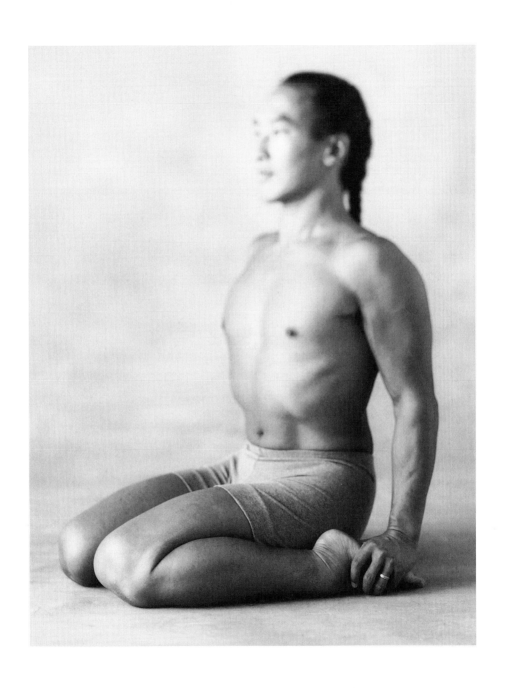

Considering the Practice

ODE TO THE ONION

Onion,
luminous flask,
your beauty formed
petal by petal,
crystal scales expanded you
and in the secrecy of the dark earth
your belly grew round with dew.
Under the earth
the miracle
happened
and when your clumsy
green stem appeared,
and your leaves were born
like swords
in the garden,
the earth heaped up her power
showing your naked transparency,
and as the remote sea
in lifting the breasts of Aphrodite
uplicated the magnolia,
so did the earth
make you,
onion,
clear as a planet,
and destined
to shine,
constant constellation,
round rose of water,
upon
the table
of the poor.

Generously
you undo
your globe of freshness
in the fervent consummation
of the cooking pot,
and the crystal shred
in the flaming heat of the oil
is transformed into a curled golden feather.

Then, too, I will recall how fertile
is your influence on the love of the salad,
and it seems that the sky contributes
by giving you the shape of hailstones
to celebrate your chopped brightness
on the hemispheres of a tomato.
But within reach
of the hands of the common people,
sprinkled with oil,
dusted
with a bit of salt,
you kill the hunger
of the day-laborer on his hard path.

Star of the poor,
fairy godmother
wrapped
in delicate
paper, you rise from the ground
eternal, whole, pure
like an astral seed,
and when the kitchen knife
cuts you, there arises
the only tear
without sorrow.

You make us cry without hurting us.
I have praised everything that exists,
but to me, onion, you are
more beautiful than a bird
of dazzling feathers,
you are to my eyes
a heavenly globe, a platinum goblet,
an unmoving dance
of the snowy anemone

and the fragrance of the earth lives
in your crystalline nature.

— PABLO NERUDA

Grounding. You are not separate from the earth; you are *of* the earth. And grounding means touching the ground, really touching it. Let the natural expression of the earth rise up through your body. And then, from that groundedness, begin to move, and to grow, just as a tree grows taller by first extending its roots.

Foundation. Your feet provide the foundation for all your standing poses. So plant your feet. Imprint them on the ground. Enmesh your feet in the earth like the shallow roots of a giant sequoia. Feel the weightedness of your entire body falling into the ground *through* your feet. For without a foundation, there can be no rising.

Standing Poses. The standing poses are the poses that teach you how to connect to the earth and draw energy up through your feet and legs into the rest of your body. Through them, you rediscover the true nature of your legs, both as roots and as movers. These poses help you align your feet and legs in relationship to your pelvis and spine, which is fundamental to integrating your entire body:

Mountain Pose

Downward-Facing Dog

Triangle Pose

Side Angle Pose

Warrior Pose 1

Warrior Pose 2

1. Staff Pose

10 to 15 breaths

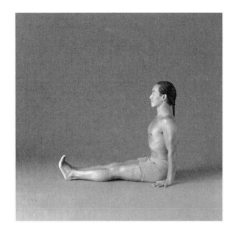

Instructions. Root the backs of your legs into the earth. Activate and open the soles of your feet by spreading your toes and stretching the skin of the soles of your feet. Place your legs so that your knees and your toes are pointing straight up toward the ceiling. Reach strongly through your heels and the balls of your feet away from your hips as you activate your arches. With your hands beside your hips, press down into the ground, elongating your waist and lifting your chest, while you maintain an ease that allows your breath to flow.

One Thing. Pulse your legs into the ground as your belly stays watery and supple, and let your torso begin to rise from the pulsations.

2. Mountain Pose

15 to 25 breaths

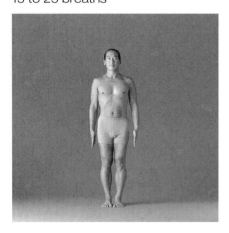

Instructions. Lift all your toes off the ground, and feel your heels, the mounds of your big toes, and the spread of your baby toes. Let your feet be like tree frog feet, sticky and tenacious. Feel the arches of your feet—the centers of your feet—rising.

Now, lay your toes back on the ground. Let the strength of your legs rise from your sensitive, active feet up to the base of your spine. Contract and draw up the fronts of your thighs, and spread your calf muscles wide as they descend toward your heel bones. From the pillars of your legs, elongate your waist into your open, expansive chest. Float your head over your chest like a pelican hanging in the sky peering down deep into the ocean, watching for a fish.

One Thing. Feel the stem of your body connecting to the earth through the roots of your legs and feet. The whole earth is underneath you.

3. Downward-Facing Dog

15 to 30 breaths
Repetitions: 1 to 2 times

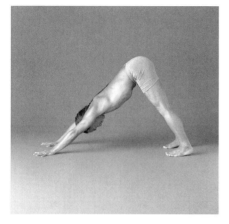

Instructions. Shift your weight from one hand to the other and from one foot to the other to find a place where your weight falls evenly into your hands and feet.

From the strength of your legs—like horses pulling back on the carriage of your body—pull your thighbones back toward your hamstrings. Let that pull of your legs be a continuous action that elongates your waist and makes you feel as if your hands have to reach to stay connected to the ground. Rest your neck and head between your arms, so the action of your arms and legs becomes unlaced from any pushing and aggressiveness of your mind.

One Thing. Extend your arms and legs from your grounded hands and feet, as if you were a plant drawing water from the earth.

4. Triangle Pose

10 to 15 breaths per side
Repetitions: 1 to 2 times (right and left, then right and left again)

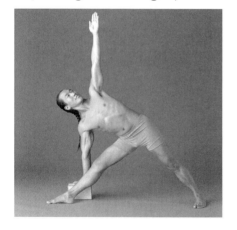

Instructions. Before turning your pelvis to shift into the pose, open your back foot—spread your toes and feel your tenacious, sticky tree frog feet. Then, as you shift into the pose, ground your back leg even more, feeling its vibrant strength digging into the earth. Your movement into the pose drives your roots even deeper into the ground. *Plummeting your heels into the earth.*

From this living foundation, extend your spine from your tailbone to the crown of your head as equally as you can between right side and left side. This should accentuate the movement in your hip socket (the part from which you want to move in this pose). Place your right hand down on your shin or on a block, keeping the strength of your legs, the openness of your chest, and the balance of your torso over the plane of your legs.

One Thing. The wide triangular base of your legs rising from your writhing feet, moving into the light of your spine.

5. Side Angle Pose

10 to 15 breaths per side
Repetitions: 1 to 2 times (right and
left, then right and left again)

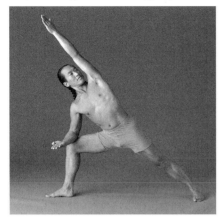

Instructions. Keep the reach of your back leg and the grounded-ness of your back foot as you bend your front leg to 90 degrees. With your right elbow on your right knee, press down to open your chest and extend your spine. Feel how your top arm carries the line of energy from your back leg through your spine into your left fingertips. *The spiral of your trunk arising from the roots of your legs moving all the way up to your head as it looks skyward.*

One Thing. This is one of the most challenging yoga poses in which to create space, so rooting your back leg is more impor-tant than ever now. Dig your feet into the ground, and muster your strength to extend your spine and turn your body to face the sun.

6. Warrior Pose 1

5 to 10 breaths per side
Repetitions: 1 to 2 times (right and
left, then right and left again)

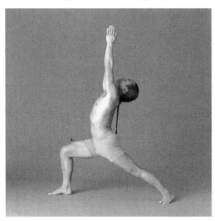

Instructions. As you turn your hips to face your front leg, feel the spiral of your pelvis and torso corkscrewing upward, from your outer back heel through the reach of your arms. Keep the dy-namic tension between your front leg, which is bending toward 90 degrees, and your back leg, which is pressing into the ground and away from the ground. The pulling and pushing between your legs funnels energy upward into your rising chest and your thrusting arms. *Let your mind abandon its determination as your head arcs upward from the bed of your heart.*

One Thing. Create one beautiful, integrated arc, from your back foot to your fingertips. Let your connection to the earth—through the rootedness of your back leg—free you from strain and struggle.

7. Warrior Pose 2

10 to 15 breaths per side
Repetitions: 1 to 2 times (right and
left, then right and left again)

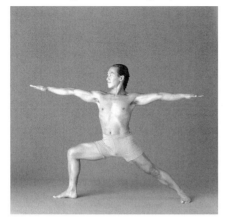

Instructions. As you come into the pose, as you sustain the pose, and as you come out of the pose, focus your attention on your back leg and back arm, making them consciously vigorous. Your back leg and back arm are the energetic foundation for the entire pose. *Pummel your heel into the ground, like crushing herbs.*

Your pelvis is a supple conduit for the energy being drawn up from your legs, so continue to search for the most effective way to draw that energy through to the channel of your spine into the blossoming of your arms. As you are gazing over your front hand, allow your vision to come into your open eyes, without reaching for it (the nature of your eyes is to see; therefore, just let the light pour into them).

One Thing. Don't lock into this pose (or any pose); be loose and responsive. The whole earth is underneath you, so ride its energy—its power—as if you were surfing a wave. Gaze over your front arm as if you were gazing toward the distant, sandy shore.

8. Reclined Leg Stretch

15 to 25 breaths per side

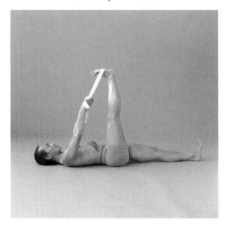

Instructions. Focus strongly on your bottom leg—on rooting it into the ground—and feel the extension of your spine. Bring your awareness to your entire back body as it rests against the earth. With so much of your body against the ground now, can you grow your top leg from that rootedness?

Use your arms to open your chest just as much as to stretch your hamstrings. As you pull with your arms, draw them back into their sockets, which will help to broaden your collarbones and lift your chest further from your pelvis. Relax your neck and head.

One Thing. Not all grounding is work. So let your whole body fall into the earth, and enhance the downward movement with your muscular effort and your mental attention. Be as open and vulnerable as a dog on its back, waiting for a belly rub.

9. Cobbler's Pose

15 to 30 breaths

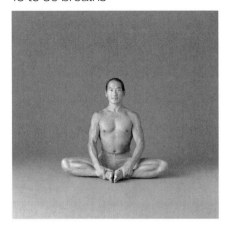

Instructions. Allow your groundedness in this pose—and your release—to come from the very tops of your thighbones falling into the ground. Let your legs spread wide on the surface of the earth, like falling rain soaking into the ground.

As you hold your ankles, pull with your arms just enough to expand and open your chest. Use your back muscles as little as possible. Instead release your groins more and more to come toward the natural curves of your spine. As you discover the resistance in your hips, try to pinpoint where that resistance is, and then let it go. Realize that grounding can come just as much from surrender as it can from effort.

One Thing. Feel the complete surrender of your legs as the roots that allow your pelvis to grow upright and your spine to rise, as if your legs are a lily pad and your spine is rising from it like the flower's stem.

10. One-Legged Forward Bend

7 to 15 breaths per side
Repetitions: 1 to 2 times (right and left, then right and left again)

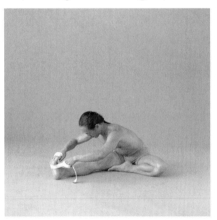

Instructions. If you cannot easily reach the foot of your extended leg, place a strap around it and hold one end of the strap in each hand. Draw forward by bending your arms. Initiate the twist and forward bend of your body from your legs. The strength of the grounding of your legs propels your chest forward and over your straight leg. *Root, rise up, twist, and release forward.*

Extend your spine so there is a continuous even arc from your tailbone to the crown of your head. Even though your torso is rounded, search for a sense of equanimity between your front and back body. Let your arms help extend your body by drawing your chest away from your pelvis, which is grounded by your legs. (If this seems to irritate your lower back at all, sit on the edge of a folded blanket and keep your spine more extended and less rounded.)

One Thing. Let the asymmetry of your foundation spiral into a release of your spine over your extended leg. Feel the unleashing of the power of your back body.

11. Seated Forward Bend
15 to 30 breaths

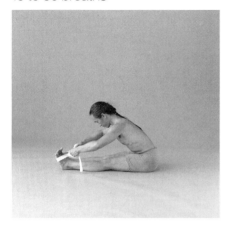

Instructions. If you cannot easily reach your feet, place a strap around them and hold one end of the strap in each hand. Draw forward by bending your arms. Press your legs down strongly to elongate your side waist. Tilt your sacrum more into a forward bend as you release your groins, so your lower back doesn't take too much pressure. Move forward toward your feet as much as you do down toward your legs. Then lift and broaden your heart and lungs, and surrender your head. *Ground, extend, fold forward, turn inward.*

Transform the density of your legs into the suppleness of your pelvis into the energy of your solar plexus into the spaciousness of your chest into the expanse of your mind. *Earth to water to fire to air to ether.* (If this seems to irritate your lower back at all, sit on the edge of a folded blanket and keep your spine more extended and less rounded.)

One Thing. Let the energy you gather from your legs rise up your back and then coil into your center. Fold onto yourself. Propel yourself inward. Create a reflection that allows you see yourself like the reflection of a full moon on a still pond.

12. Reclined Cobbler's Pose
3 to 5 minutes

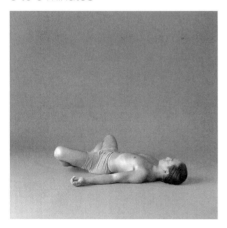

Instructions. Drop your legs, release your groins, and allow your belly to be receptive. Make any minute adjustments that allow your back body to be broader, longer, and more at ease on the ground. Let your mind continue to feel more and more subtle connections to the earth. Feel how your breath itself rises from and returns to the ground. Your exhalations especially teach you how to trust and surrender.

One Thing. Surrender the seed of your body into the earth, water it, and let it blossom.

13. Relaxation Pose

5 to 10 minutes

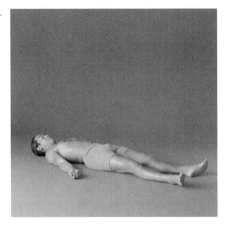

Instructions. Your entire body is planted on and supported by the earth—let yourself surrender completely. *Make a breath print on the earth.*

One Thing. Let go of separateness—of the illusion of separateness—and of the boundaries of your individual consciousness. Be held in the arms of mother earth. *Complete surrender. Complete restoration.*

14. Sitting Meditation

5 minutes or intuition

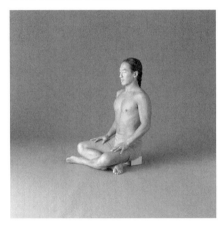

Sitting. Let your hips come back to their natural openness by sitting in a simple crossed-legged position. Feel the root of your spine, along with your legs, connecting to the earth.

Meditating. Sit and feel your connectedness to the earth—

> *your posture rising from the fluidity of your spine—*
> *the ease with which you can balance over your*
> *connectedness—*
> *the small finger of your individual existence on the huge*
> *body of the planet*

Can you let your mind broaden into a much larger consciousness, supported by your contact with the ground?

Reconsidering the Practice

Do you remember as a child lying on the lawn looking up at the sky and feeling the whole wide-open summer in front of you as you watched the clouds moving, forming, and re-forming? How the summer grass was the perfect support for your body and yet sometimes awakened you by scratching and tickling and poking your skin? How all your worries seemed to drop away and you felt so free?

And do you remember that sometimes when things got difficult, just going outside and walking barefoot in the dirt, climbing a tree, or swimming in the river could make your problems seem smaller and less significant?

Our bodies and our minds are still of that nature—they still get relief from being connected to the earth. But as adults, most of us get so far removed from that connection. We walk around the world in rubber-soled shoes on concrete sidewalks, which insulate us from any contact with unevenness, irregularity, or unpredictability. And our feet, which are one of the most sensitive parts of our bodies, are locked up in their pretty little boxes. So even when you aren't doing yoga, you can still take off your shoes, rub your feet, soak them in warm water, and have a friend massage them and caress them.

Then you can walk around in your house and actually feel everything you step on: the satiny warmth of a hardwood floor, the rough nubbiness of a carpet, the cold brittleness of tile. You can even go into nature without your shoes on. Step on smooth sand and sharp rocks and slimy mud and crispy dry leaves—just walk down the trail.

Because what other ground is there for you to stand on? Isn't the rest of it—your ideals, your beliefs, your work, your family, your friends—merely quicksand?

Grounding Practice Summary

1. Staff Pose
10 to 15 breaths

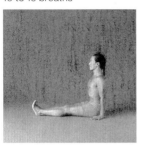

2. Mountain Pose
15 to 25 breaths

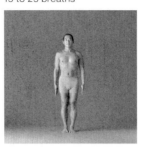

3. Downward-Facing Dog
15 to 30 breaths, 1 to 2 times

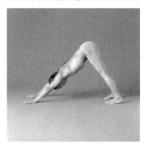

4. Triangle Pose
10 to 15 breaths per side, 1 to 2 times

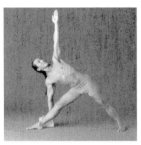

5. Side Angle Pose
10 to 15 breaths per side, 1 to 2 times

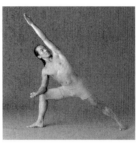

6. Warrior Pose 1
5 to 10 breaths per side, 1 to 2 times

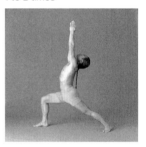

7. Warrior Pose 2
10 to 15 breaths per side, 1 to 2 times

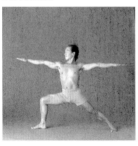

8. Reclined Leg Stretch
15 to 25 breaths per side

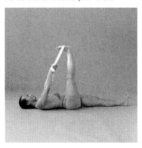

9. Cobbler's Pose
15 to 30 breaths

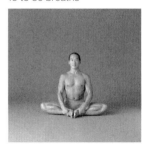

10. One-Legged Forward Bend

7 to 15 breaths per side,
1 to 2 times

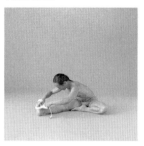

11. Seated Forward Bend

15 to 30 breaths

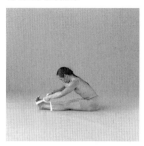

12. Reclined Cobbler's Pose

3 to 5 minutes

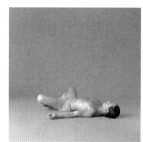

13. Relaxation Pose

5 to 10 minutes

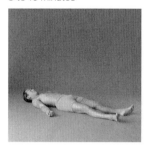

14. Sitting Meditation

5 minutes or intuition

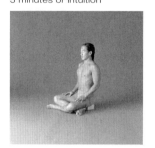

NONSTOP

What if the flight from Boston to San Francisco really did take forever and the captain came on the intercom and announced, "Well, folks, I've got some good news and some bad news: the bad news is that the earth has disappeared from sight and no longer registers on our instruments, and so it seems that we are stranded here in the sky for all eternity, in a luminous, cloudy limbo somewhere between our original point of departure and our scheduled destination, and the good news is that there is an endless supply of fuel as well as complimentary beverages and meals—miraculously, our supplies completely replenish themselves after each usage, somewhat like that bottomless pitcher of wine in the ancient Greek myth—so at least we won't be contemplating cannibalism or taking a sudden dive into an unknown void—and frankly, I'm hoping that there might be a member of the clergy on board, or a philosopher, or even a scientist, who could help us all deal with the predicament in which we have found ourselves because, I confess, I am at a total loss," would the passenger doing crossword puzzles in seat 21E volunteer to take a shift as a stewardess, and ask the name of each person to whom she served a meal on a plastic tray, saying "So glad to meet you" in a warm, gentle voice with a southern accent, and would the passenger hunched over his laptop in seat 14B close his spreadsheet and begin writing about his childhood on the coast of Maine instead, and would the passenger wearing headphones in seat 25A turn off her CD player and take her flute down from the overhead bin and, when everyone got tired and the shades were pulled down to simulate night, begin to play a mysterious, haunting tune, and would I stop reading, tucking my book into the seat pocket in front of me, and pull my son, who is on the verge of becoming too old for such things, onto my lap and simply hold him there, reveling in the tender-heavy weight of his long limbs, the glistening fur-feel of his razor-cut boy-hair, the unblemished nectarine skin of his summer-sunburned cheek, the cinnamon-vanilla-coffee scent of his neck?

— NINA ZOLOTOW

Why We Do Yoga, Part 2

NINA   I just wanted to ask you about how you got started. I know a lot of people look at you and think you're so flexible that it must have been easy for you. They see you where you are now, and they have no idea how you were when you started.

ROD   I've been practicing yoga for about twenty years at this point. I started in 1980, and I got into yoga because I was very tight both physically and emotionally. I think at that point in my life I was becoming very sad and very disappointed that a lot of my idealism was being crushed, by being in college and by being in my early twenties. I think that I was very sad because what people call "the real world" was descending on my dreams. And I felt the weight of that. It was like a really dark cloud that was going to envelop me and devour me for the rest of my life. I remember taking my first yoga class because I was a ballet dancer, and I was still very inflexible, and a friend and I used to so-called stretch before and after every ballet class, but with some success and with some frustration. We weren't really getting as open and flexible as we wanted to. And there was a yoga studio right above the dance studio and so we took a class, and I still vividly remember how I felt after that first class.

   More than anything what I remember is feeling emotionally balanced and cleansed. I felt really unbound by my past and unbound by expectations, and I felt really alive—that is what yoga did for me in the early years. It was an unbinding of a lot of the restrictions that I was placing on myself from growing up in a family—you know, like everybody—and having certain relationships with my parents—having a really tumultuous, argumentative relationship with my father—having sort of a secret pact with my mother that I would be safe. Yoga brought me to a place where I could listen to what my parents had to say—I could listen to their concerns—but I was no longer bound by the silent agreements that we had made.

NINA   All from one class?

ROD   Well, no, but for the first three years of yoga, that's what yoga meant to me. First of all, I was already used to practicing a lot because I was a ballet dancer, so I immediately took on the practice of yoga strongly. And I think because of that, its power to affect me was very strong. And for the first three years, I felt like the reason I was practicing was that every time I practiced, I felt a freedom. I felt an amazing sense of being able to breathe—really being able to breathe—and being light in my step and having a sense of hope again (which is something I don't actually believe in now so much—the idea of hope—but at that point I think it inspired me to examine my life more deeply). But now I want to ask you, why did *you* start yoga?

NINA   I started it by accident. It was at work, and there was some empty space in the office building, and we talked about having an exercise class there, and one of the men who worked there said that his wife could teach it. And so she came to teach us. I didn't even know that I was doing yoga, and . . . I had studied ballet as a child—this is something I haven't told you yet. I loved it, but I was really bad at it.

ROD   You loved ballet?

NINA   Yes, I loved ballet. I loved it, but I was really bad at it. And everyone discouraged me. I was always at the bottom of the class. And there was one point when they put everyone in the class on toe except me—which was cruel—but I still hung in there. And then the teachers were all saying to my mother, you know, "Your daughter has absolutely no talent for this, no natural flexibility, no strength," no whatever.

ROD   But isn't it amazing? You know, when I look back at my dance years, I think that at least ballet gave me a deep appreciation for my body, even though it was really judgmental.

NINA   Yes. I felt some connection to it, that's all I can say. But it was just wrong, the wrong thing for me. So then in this yoga class when we got to stand with our feet straight instead of turned out, I was so happy. And all of a sudden I felt like, "Oh, I can do this!" It felt right.

ROD You know, that's the funny thing—I've talked to a lot of people who were ridiculed in their PE classes and also in sports and so forth, and when they come to yoga, they actually feel like they've found something they can approach without someone coming down on them as if they had some foreign, alien body. And also, in a yoga class, even if there are different levels in one class, there is for most people a much more noncompetitive aspect to yoga, where people can be in their bodies and not feel inadequate.

NINA Yes. It's the same story for me. I wasn't very good at sports and always got picked—well, not the last because I was fairly popular, but they would pick all the good people and then they would start picking the people they liked, so then I would get picked [laughs]. They wanted to make sure to beef up the team with people who could actually play first. And I always had this image of myself as someone who wasn't physical and who was cerebral and all that. But anyway, I just took classes for a couple of years, and then I started getting more into it—

ROD What do you mean by "started getting more into it"?

NINA I started feeling like I wanted to do more. I didn't really have a strong idea of why. I told Mary the other day that my metaphor for my relationship with yoga now is that it has been like looking at the boy next door and realizing you've been in love the whole time but that it took all those years to get there.

ROD So it was just something you were doing—you just kept on going back to it because it was something that felt sort of right. And then all of a sudden you just realized how much you really liked it, how much it was really a part of you, and how much it did for you, maybe. So why do you do it now, many years later?

NINA I have so many feelings. Partly I just really enjoy it now. I enjoy doing it, and when I start practicing I start trying to find excuses to make it last longer. But that sounds crazy. I know some people want to . . .

ROD . . . get through it.

NINA But because of my family and everything I am supposed to be doing, I'm thinking, well, it's a quarter to six, I really should be cooking dinner, but maybe I could just sneak in a headstand. . . . Then Brad comes home and he says, "What's for dinner?"

ROD   That's why your husband's gotten good at cooking, I see.

NINA   He gets a little annoyed sometimes, because he's been at work, and he walks in the door, and what he wants is the smell of food and everybody there waiting for him at the table, but instead he's got me doing a headstand.

But anyway, yoga just feels really good. I have had some little fantasies about it, that it might help me sleep better or help me feel calmer in certain situations, but I don't think those fantasies are what motivates me to do it. I would be doing it anyway, even if I knew those things would *never* happen.

ROD   You know what's really interesting—as you're talking, I'm thinking about the one thing that really shifted for me during all these years. When I was a ballet dancer, I had a really poor image of myself. This was partly because I didn't have a typical ballet body (that is, a short torso with a long neck, arms, and legs). And partly because I wasn't quite coordinated or rhythmical enough. Furthermore, I was an Asian male practicing a Eurocentric art form.

NINA   You couldn't dance for the San Francisco Ballet because you didn't *look* right.

ROD   I didn't have "the look." And you know what? I have to say that after somewhere around ten years of yoga, I started really liking my body. I mean I started really appreciating it for what it was and what it could do and—and even appreciating it for what it couldn't do. As if the things that I was learning from the resistance of my body were really exciting. And I actually began to appreciate my difficulties and also my beauties, and what I used to consider the elements that made me into the ugly duckling I became fond of through yoga, interestingly enough. I became fond of my idiosyncrasies and my uniqueness. So actually that's what I want to ask you about. I know for me, yoga really changed my body image. And you were saying how you were sort of like the person—not quite the last being picked on the teams, but in ballet class you were the one that was the least promising . . .

NINA   The last one to go on toe.

ROD   So did yoga really change your body image?

NINA   Yes. What's changed for me is that I never thought of myself as being strong at all. I'm small and small boned, and with yoga I've learned how to do things in my forties that I could never do in my life.

ROD   Like handstand?

NINA   Yes, handstand, and long headstands, elbow balance, and, you know, I'm starting to be able to do the arm balances. Have you seen me there in the back? I've been having so much fun.

ROD   So it does ring true that—I mean as yoga teachers we actually say that if you learn these arm balances, you'll gain a new sense of self-confidence. And I've never had to do that personally because I've actually been really strong in my upper body, so I've just sort of said that because I thought that it might happen. But you're actually experiencing that.

NINA   Yes. And to me it's very metaphorical. It makes me feel like a stronger person.

ROD   To be able to be on your arms?

NINA   Learning to do handstand took me so long. I could do it if someone helped me up, but I was terrified of going up by myself. My heart would drop into my throat. So when I first started to kick up into a handstand by myself, no matter what bad things were happening, I felt like I had this little talisman: "But I can do handstands!"

ROD   You know, I can't tell you how many women have called me at strange times during the night screaming in my phone, "I got up in a handstand by myself!" It's a profound thing to accomplish something that you would never have even dreamed of doing, especially at this time in your life.

NINA   Exactly. There used to be a woman in my yoga class who could do hand-stand—she had learned it when she was young—and then she left the class. And one day I ran into her, and she asked, "Have you gotten up in a handstand yet?" And I said, "No." And she said, "Well, you know, maybe you're just too old. Maybe it's just *never* going to happen." [laughs].

ROD   You're too old.

NINA   I'd love to see her again. "Hi!"

ROD   "Check this out."

NINA   That's right.

ROD   So you've been taking class for a while and you've had a lot of different teachers and so forth, and maybe you've done some reading on yoga, or maybe you've read every popular book there is because you have to write this book. But what I'm curious about is, what have you gotten out of all this education? What do you feel are some of the basic tenets of yoga, maybe just one or two things that come to mind?

NINA   I have a real hard time with that because—

ROD   Well, that's good. Let's go into it.

NINA   —because I'm very skeptical about a lot of the things people say, even a lot of things that you say.

ROD   [laughs] Like what?

NINA   So what I'm trying to do is just go along for the ride and see what happens. I'm trying not to have my own ideas about what yoga is, and I'm trying to just see what happens as I go along.

ROD   What's the purpose of skepticism?

NINA   My sister-in-law once said something very interesting about me. She said, "Nina's not shy, but she's very protected."

ROD   So skepticism protects you, maybe?

NINA   Yes. That's not something I worked out in advance of this conversation, but—

ROD   No, I think that's really a good free association. That's profound.

NINA   Thank you, teacher [sardonically]. So what I've decided to do is to try to suspend my skepticism and just go along on the journey with you and everybody else, my other teachers and the other students, and see what happens. So that's why I'm reluctant to say, "Oh, yoga's this, or yoga's that." But that's me. I can just be doing it because I'm attracted to it.

ROD   That's right.

NINA   And I don't need to believe it, or in it.

ROD   You don't really need a reason.

NINA   Right. Here's a little story about that. Every once in a while I "detach." This
        means that I stand in class and I look at what everybody's doing, and I sud-
        denly think, "What am I doing here with these people? They're all staring at
        this one guy's body, and he's moving this one little muscle, and this is com-
        pletely crazy. . . ." Well, one night—after having had one of those moments
        during a class—I e-mailed my friend Melitta, who had missed the class, and
        after telling her what the class had been like, I wrote in all capital letters,
        WHY DO I EVEN DO THIS STUFF? And she e-mailed back, "We do yoga be-
        cause it makes our lives better." And ever since then, that's been it.

ROD   Your little phrase.

NINA   Yes. That, to me, is just basic enough.

ROD   Actually, I totally agree with that. I think that all the things that your teach-
        ers say are basically expounding on that fact. Why does yoga make my life
        better? What is it actually doing? And why do I feel better after yoga class?
        Why does my body feel much more harmonious? What is my mind and
        emotional state? It's just a furthering of that statement, really. If you gener-
        ally asked everybody that question of why they do yoga, I think really their
        root answer is "Yoga basically makes my life better." As someone who's been
        trying to explain it to a lot of different people and who is also questioning
        myself about my own practice, I, too, get to that same question: "What the
        hell am I doing?" You know, there are a lot of things to do in the world—a lot
        of interesting things to see and do and cultures to deal with—

NINA   Yes, because let's say you're in Hawaii and it's gorgeous, and then you're in
        this room with these people, and they're all looking at their feet or some-
        thing—

ROD   Yes, you might just want to lie on the ground and look up. But—see—the
        thing is that a lot of times, we can be in a really beautiful place and still be
        in our heads, you know? And then we can't actually be in that beautiful
        place.

NINA   What are we doing right now?

ROD   No, I'm not in my head. I'm looking at you. Looking at you and with the blue backdrop. But here's a good example: I used to teach a Friday night class and no one else could build up that class. It was at the Yoga Room in Berkeley. And it sort of started slowly—the class didn't build immediately. But when people started realizing what yoga was doing for them—creating a reprieve between their workweek and their weekend—they started feeling that they were free to enjoy Friday, Saturday, and Sunday, when most people take until Sunday morning before they can really drop into the weekend.

   And for me, it has become more like that. Yes, I may be scheduled to fly to Texas to teach yoga, or I might be in the classroom teaching yoga, but because of the practice, there's a sense of freedom, or dimension of freedom, that is: yes, I am here now and this is what I'm doing, and I'm fine and I'm alive. And then it doesn't really matter—I can be looking up at the sky or I can be looking at a ceiling that's two feet away from my face. And yet I'm alive in the world and I'm living my life. I'm not fantasizing about my life or I'm not in some illusion in my head and then someday I'm going to wake up and say, "Oh, my God! What did I ever really see? Who did I ever really touch? Who did I ever really talk to?"

AN ALIGNMENT PRACTICE

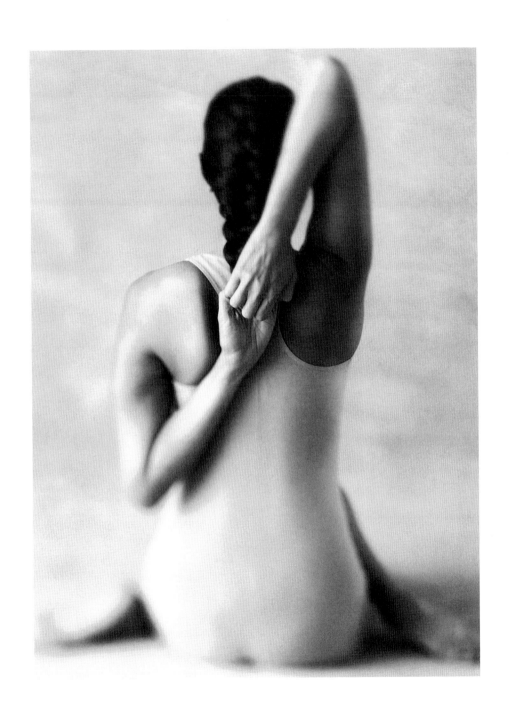

Considering the Practice

Alignment. The deeper the alignment of your pose is, the less effort you need. And the more you refine your alignment around center, the closer you come to true balance. *A natural, organic alignment.* Like a six-month-old baby sitting for the first time, using gentle movements, bringing itself to center over its skeletal structure.

> *gross alignment*
> *to refined alignment*
> *to observation and response*
> *to coordination between all body parts*
> *to freedom of breath*

Bones. Bones can carry the weight of the body so the muscles can be supple for freedom of movement and circulation. (If you were a boneless animal, you would be just slithering on the ground.) Downward-Facing Dog is a good example. When your elbows and shoulders are lined up, your weight is carried by your bones. If your arms are bent, your muscles are holding up the pose.

Muscles. This practice will help your muscles become more supple so you will have more freedom of movement. Your circulation will be enhanced, your muscles moving more easily from contraction to deep relaxation and vice versa. Yoga will help with the coordination of your body, enabling you to fire and relax the appropriate muscles.

Centering. Each limb and each part of your body has a center—an important aspect of alignment. So can you bear your weight in your center, with the force of your muscle in the center of your limb? For example, in Mountain Pose, can you align your weight in the front of your heel, in the center of your body? Alignment—like centering—is a dialogue. So listen, play, feel, change, and listen again.

Relaxing. Many positions work energetically in your body. So consider not only your skeletal structure but also how deeply you can relax in any given pose. For relaxation without collapse creates a pure conduit for the life force. Be precise and hone your sense of alignment, but this means searching for an *organic* alignment, not a symmetrical alignment.

Alignment Poses. The following poses allow you to explore alignment in standing, seated, twisting, back-bending, forward-bending, and reclined positions:

Mountain Pose

Standing Forward Bend

Triangle Pose

Warrior Pose 2

Sideways Extension Pose

Downward-Facing Dog

Hero Pose

Bridge Pose

Marichi's Pose

Wide-Angle Forward Bend

Reclined Leg Stretch

Relaxation Pose

Cobbler's Pose

1. Mountain Pose

15 to 30 breaths

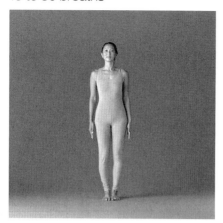

Instructions. Stand in Mountain Pose and gaze at your profile in the mirror. Where is the plumb line?

center of your ear over
center of your shoulder over
center of your hip over
center of your leg over
center of your heel

Now stand in Mountain Pose and gaze at the front of your body in the mirror. Where is the plumb line?

center of your head over
center of your chest over
center of your pelvis over
center of your legs over
center of your heels

Are both knees aligned with both feet, both shoulders aligned with each other, and both sides of the waist of equal length?

One Thing. Can you feel your skeleton? Can you begin to orient yourself off the feeling of your skeleton? To play around with the relationship of the different bones?

Play with different sensations. And try to realize that a lot of times what feels right is just your habit. Perfect alignment doesn't exist, but there is always a deeper, more intimate conversation. Play with feeling the weight of your head right over your heart and lungs, over the core of your body. How is the weight falling on your feet? Is it even?

2. Standing Forward Bend
10 to 15 breaths

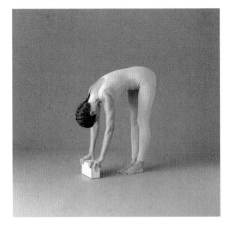

Instructions. Align yourself so that your kneecaps are lifting and aligned over your second and third toes. Feel the backs of your thighs drawn up as much as the fronts, the insides of your legs drawn up as much as the outsides. Look at your feet and see how the weight is falling on them.

For most people, alignment in this pose does not mean being straight up and down; instead, the feeling of letting your weight fall evenly into your feet is what is important. Allow your spine to hang in a gentle, released curve, as evenly as possible, like a waterfall pouring from the height of your sitting bones and over the earth of your legs.

One Thing. Search for an alignment of your spine that creates an equanimity of surrender throughout your body.

3. Triangle Pose
10 to 15 breaths per side
Repetitions: 1 to 2 times (right and left, then right and left again)

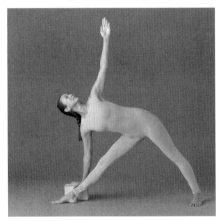

Instructions. Align yourself so that the heel of your front foot is lined up with the heel of your back foot. Make sure your front kneecap points in the direction of the third toe of your front foot and that your torso is in the plane of your front leg. The emphasis in this pose is not in how far you come down over your front leg but in finding the integrity of the alignment of your spine, which stems from the evenness of the work of both your legs.

One Thing. Search for an alignment where your skeleton feels open, where your joints and your skeleton—especially at the shoulders—don't feel jammed. Search for a broadness in your legs and thighs moving away from each other. And see if you can find a broadness in your collarbones and shoulder blades, reaching into the arms. Extend your spine evenly on both right and left sides.

4. Standing Forward Bend
10 to 15 breaths

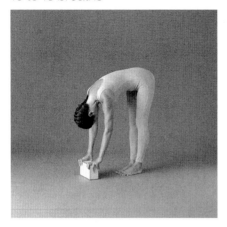

One Thing. As you repeat this pose, focus on releasing the back of your neck as your shoulder blades draw slightly up toward your pelvis. Let your head dangle completely.

5. Warrior Pose 2
10 to 15 breaths per side
Repetitions: 1 to 2 times (right and left, then right and left again)

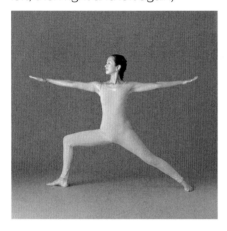

Instructions. Align yourself so that as you bend your front leg, your shinbone does not go farther than perpendicular with the ground. Your bent knee should be externally rotated from the lift of your instep. And both knees should rotate away from each other. Distribute the weight of your torso evenly between both feet by drawing your torso farther over your back leg through the reach of your back arm.

> *center of your head over*
> *center of your pelvis over*
> *center of your feet*

One Thing. Play with shifting your pelvis over the foundation of your legs, and gravitate toward whatever feels organically aligned.

6. Sideways Extension Pose

10 to 15 breaths per side
Repetitions: 1 to 2 times (right and
left, then right and left again)

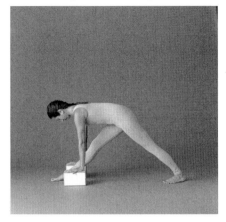

Instructions. Align yourself so your hips are as square as possible. Line up your knees with your feet, so your legs are shafts of light coming from the sun of your pelvis, your toes like a prism, a spray of light. Your weight should fall right down those shafts. The intention of your back leg should emanate from your belly through your leg down into your heels and the splay of your toes.

Try shifting the weight of the pose—your pelvis and your torso—to get evenness through your legs into your feet. Once you have the triangular foundation, cascade your spine over your front leg toward your front foot.

One Thing. Search for the deep surrender that comes from the refinement of your alignment. Your body intuitively lets go when there is truthfulness to your form, like planets aligning. Something we're innately drawn to. Listen deeply to the call of your body, its natural call to be aligned and at ease.

7. Standing Forward Bend

10 to 15 breaths

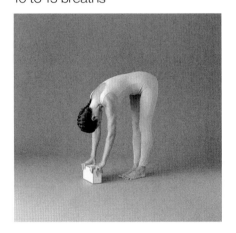

One Thing. As you repeat this pose, focus on breathing into your back body, as your back muscles spread wide from your spine. Let your breath be your guide to alignment.

8. Downward-Facing Dog

15 to 30 breaths

Repetitions: 1 to 2 times

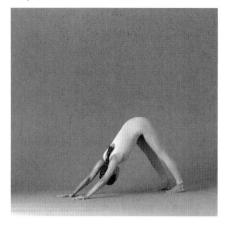

Instructions. Align your ankles, your knees, and your hip joints so that the weight of your body is carried evenly through the supporting columns of your legs. Wiggle your pelvis, torso, and arms, feeling their skeletal alignment, and then place them as best you can in one direct line from sitting bones to fingertips. Center your lower ribs so the drape of your skin feels even along your torso.

> *heels to sitting bones*
> *sitting bones to fingertips—*
> *waist long*
> *ribs centered*

One Thing. The truer your alignment, the more even your feet and hands will be on the ground. So keep looking, searching, and listening.

9. Hero Pose

15 to 30 breaths

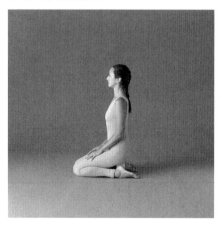

Instructions. Align yourself so the soles of your feet are directly up toward the ceiling, keeping the top of your feet and center of your shinbones on the ground. Sit on a prop that is high enough so your pelvis can be upright with a natural curve in your lower back. As you release your groins, rotate your thighs away from each other. Be lifted, open, and attentive.

> *center of head over*
> *center of chest over*
> *center of pelvis over*
> *center of earth*

One Thing. Search for a rising up from the deep surrender and gravity of your legs. Can you find a strong buoyancy from their density?

10. Bridge Pose

10 to 15 breaths

Repetitions: 1 to 2 times

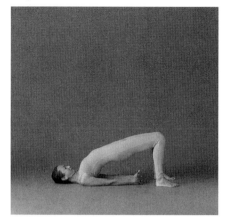

Instructions. Align yourself so that your are feet are parallel and hips-distance apart. Drop your knees slightly toward each other—don't let them splay outward. Feel the strength of your legs pressing evenly into your feet. Let your neck stay passive—your chest moving up toward the ceiling from the grounding of your arms, sacrum floating upward as your lower back lengthens.

You can't utilize the true power of your legs without alignment. It is the alignment of your legs that allows the flow of *prana*—the breath. So see if you can use the strength of your legs as a supportive part of your body rather than as an aggressive part of your body. Your sensitivity will come from feeling your feet, your knees, and your hip joints—and how they are coordinating with each other. Then the work of your legs can give you a true opening of your chest.

Can you build a beautiful arc with your body, like an arched doorway made of perfectly chosen stones?

> *knees aligning over feet*
> *pelvis rising to meet chest*
> *chest opening to receive*
> *arms rolling under to lift chest*
> *head resting softly*

One Thing. Without alignment you get brute force and hardness, so search for the skeletal structure of this pose. Don't jam or thrust your chest toward your head. As your front body is lifting, see if you can let your back body feel elongated. Let your front body be receptive and supported.

11. Marichi's Pose 1

10 to 15 breaths per side
Repetitions: 1 to 2 times (right and
left, then right and left again)

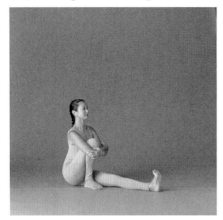

Instructions. Align yourself so that both sides of your body get an even lift, even though your legs are in different positions. Extend your straight leg strongly. Press the foot of your bent leg on the ground, keeping your knee right over the front of your heel. Even though there is some asymmetry in your pelvis, search for symmetry by dropping your bent leg hip crease even deeper. And let your arms help harness energy upward so your chest blossoms and rises.

Channel your rib cage further into center as it towers over your hips. From this centering, elongate your waist. The alignment of asymmetry:

> *feet fanning open*
> *legs rooting downward*
> *pelvis emerging upright*
> *arms drawing into sockets*
> *chest opening broadly*

Search for ways to make Marichi's Pose 1 feel harmonious. Feel the alignment internally. See if you can find a congruous energy, a rising and stacking energy:

> *from the arches of your feet*
> *from the grounding of your thighs*
> *from the uprightness of your pelvis*
> *from the billowing of your chest*
> *from the gathering of your arms*

One Thing. Search for an energetic evenness in the confines of structural asymmetry. Your bent leg side is always shorter in a physical, structural sense, so you will need to focus more on that side to elongate. *Core alignment.* There is always a center. Even if that center is always changing. Alignment is moving into that center, *falling* into that center. Like our internal alignment in everyday life, when things are so rarely even and calm, when so often there is physical or emotional or mental contortion.

12. Wide-Angle Forward Bend
15 to 30 breaths

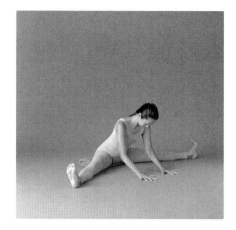

Instructions. Align yourself so that the backs of your legs contact as much of the ground as possible—moment by moment—heels, calves, hamstrings, and sitting bones. Remember being a kid and using Silly Putty to pull comic strips off the newspaper?

Look at the alignment of your legs. Are your feet vertical, with even extension on both sides of your ankles? Are the centers of both knees pointing straight up?

One Thing. Search for a stable and secure alignment in your legs as your body spills forward. The alignment of your spine *depends* on the tenacious grounding of your legs. The more your legs are aligned, the more they will be grounded, and from that grounding you can generate a great force of energy to align your spine—the way forcing water through a hose straightens the hose. The arches of your feet draw into your pelvis, your pelvis funnels energy upward, and your spine elongates with that energy into your head. *Ding!*

13. Reclined Leg Stretch
15 to 25 breaths per side

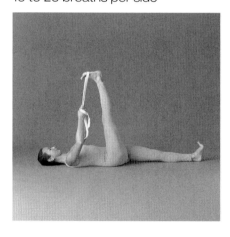

Instructions. Look at your top leg, and feel as if that foot is holding up the ceiling. Align yourself so that your knee is completely straight and yet not jammed. Then, as in the previous pose, press your top leg away, letting the thighbones of both your legs move into the flesh of your hamstrings. Draw your arms into the sockets to expand your chest. Elongate both sides of your waist evenly.

Observe the touch of your back body on the earth, and play around with feeling your bones. Move *out* of alignment to feel more what is *in* alignment.

One Thing. The articulation of one part of your body changes the alignment of your entire body. As you change the position of your foot, see if you can feel the shift resonate throughout your skeleton.

14. Relaxation Pose
5 to 10 minutes

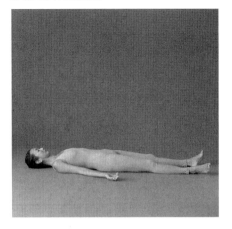

Instructions. Your body naturally relaxes more completely when there is a refined alignment. Relaxation Pose is an evenly distributed, weight-bearing pose. Your contact with the floor—your sense of touch—the knuckles of your hand, your shoulder blades, your pelvis—helps you sense your alignment. Consciously relax into symmetry, allowing for the natural curves of your spine.

One Thing. Sometimes what we sense as alignment is merely our habit, our insidious habit. And letting go into a different alignment can be disconcerting. So while you are finding that alignment, continue to bring yourself back to observing the contact of your body with the ground. This releases your agitation and allows your body to drop into a responsive, balanced alignment.

15. Sitting Meditation
5 minutes or intuition

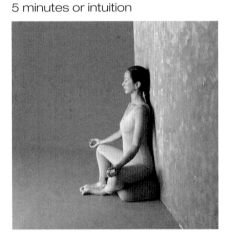

Sitting. Sit in Cobbler's Pose against a wall, with support under your legs (folded blankets or blocks). Use the wall to get feedback about the alignment of your spine, keeping your lower back slightly away from the wall and your middle back against the wall. Open your chest, with your collarbones broad and lifted from your sternum.

> *sacrum* against *the wall*
> > *lower back* away *from the wall*
> > > *middle back and shoulder blades* against *the wall*
> > > > *neck* away *from the wall*
> > > > > *back of your skull* against *the wall*

(If you wish to meditate longer than five minutes, move out of Cobbler's Pose and assume any sitting pose.)

Meditating. Observe your breath as your undulation *is* your stillness. A continual responsiveness to your alignment, like a water lily floating on a lily pond. Suspended in the movement. The flower of your breath.

Reconsidering the Practice

When things are aligned, you tend to feel a sense of ease and flow. For instance, when you're aligned mentally with someone, conversation is usually easy, both in talking and listening—so a lot gets communicated. When you feel this mental ease, there's also a change in the physical alignment of your body. For instance, you tend to be more centered in your body. When things are not aligned, you tend to feel awkward and uncomfortable. If you are eager or aggressive, you tend to be forward of the natural center of your body. If you are anxious or shy, you tend to be retracted in back of center.

So next time you find yourself in a conversation, play with changing the alignment of your body, leaning toward or away from the person, to the left or to the right, and feel how the whole conversation changes because of the alignment of your body.

And when you are out of alignment with your environment, ask yourself what is keeping you there. Is it duty? Is it fear? Is it your beliefs? Is it the need to be rebellious? Is it the need to stand out? Is it the sincere revolt of your stomach? You can't always be aligned with your environment, nor is it necessarily desirable. However, you can use your mental and physical abilities to be present. For a moment, let go of your obsessions with the past, of your likes and dislikes, and of your worries about the future, and simply observe what is. Listen, play, feel, change, and listen again. Maybe this will allow you to act with authenticity.

Alignment Practice Summary

1. Mountain Pose
15 to 30 breaths

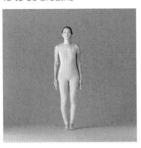

2. Standing Forward Bend
10 to 15 breaths

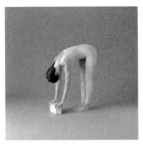

3. Triangle Pose
10 to 15 breaths per side, 1 to 2 times

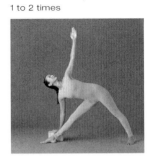

4. Standing Forward Bend
10 to 15 breaths

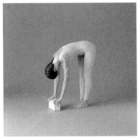

5. Warrior Pose 2
10 to 15 breaths per side, 1 to 2 times

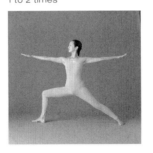

6. Sideways Extension Pose
10 to 15 breaths per side, 1 to 2 times

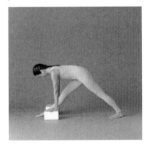

7. Standing Forward Bend
10 to 15 breaths

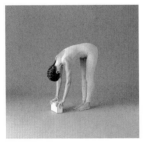

8. Downward-Facing Dog
15 to 30 breaths, 1 to 2 times

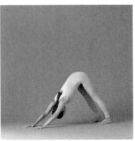

9. Hero Pose
15 to 30 breaths

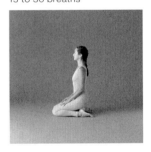

10. Bridge Pose
10 to 15 breaths, 1 to 2 times

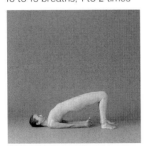

11. Marichi's Pose 1
10 to 15 breaths per side, 1 to 2 times

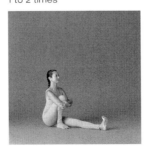

12. Wide-Angle Forward Bend
15 to 30 breaths

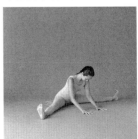

13. Reclined Leg Stretch
15 to 25 breaths per side

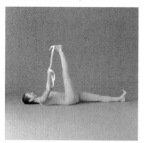

14. Relaxation Pose
5 to 10 minutes

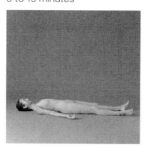

13. Sitting Meditation
5 minutes or intuition

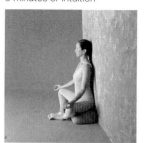

SOME CLUES ABOUT WHO I AM

More than anything, I want you to know who I really am, but that is something my parents do not allow (when I was born, my father was so ashamed of me—a monster, he called me—that he erected the endless false and misleading walls which now enclose me to ensure that he would never again have to see me, and as for my mother, it seemed that all I was to her was a constant visible reminder of her past failings, and she did not protest when I was hidden away), and so my entire life has been spent cowering here, alone in the dark, consumed by my hungers and longing for the time when you find your way to the heart of my labyrinth, for when at last you stand to meet me, face-to-face, in that all-too-brief moment before you slay me—as your own nature says you must—I will feel such an unbridled rapture, as if Aphrodite herself were embracing me on her perfumed couch, her smooth limbs as pale as alabaster, because for the first time there will be someone who sees exactly who I am but who does not turn from me and flee, and that will be as close to love as I will ever get.

Answer: the Minotaur

—NINA ZOLOTOW

Why We Do Yoga, Part 3

ROD   For me there was an immediate emotional component to the practice of yoga. When I started practicing yoga, I felt like I was no longer ruled by my emotions. I felt like I still *had* emotions—very strong emotions—in fact, I could observe them more deeply—but I felt like I was no longer controlled by them, that I actually had a sense of choice and a sense of deeper understanding because I wasn't so emotionally reactive in my life.

NINA   You said "immediate." You took one class and you felt that way?

ROD   I felt that way literally after one class, but it really had its effect over about five years. I felt immediate effects on an emotional level because of the physical balance that I felt. But on a deeper level, my emotional history began to shift. I felt like some of the things that I'd always stumbled on or got mad at or reacted to—that I actually had chances of listening and chances of being more neutral so that I could listen and observe instead of just react. But my question to you is: is there, at this point, any emotional component to yoga?

NINA   You know that I'm not as certain about it as you are. I don't feel big, dramatic changes yet.

ROD   Well, that's okay, but I'm asking you just to be straightforward. I'm not asking you to be certain. I'm asking, do you feel some emotional shifting?

NINA   No, no, Rodney, I'm trying to be honest! I *don't* feel emotionally balanced. I felt unbalanced before starting yoga, and I still feel unbalanced, really. But I believe I feel some subtle changes, and I don't know whether it's coming from the physical practice or from just being around the yoga philosophy. But I feel I'm slowly moving toward not being completely swept away by my emotions, by panic, by anxiety, by things like that. But for me, it's not like I went into my first class—or after my first five years—and then felt emotionally balanced. Also, my practice has been developing more slowly than yours did. It's been a number of years, but it hasn't been a number of years that I've been practicing intensively. Maybe if I had been practicing intensively the whole seven years, there would be something more dramatic—

ROD   How do you feel after yoga class?

NINA   I usually feel good.

ROD   When you say you feel good, what does that mean?

NINA   My body feels good, and I often feel more optimistic than I might have felt during the day. A little more optimistic, a little more cheerful. I always want to eat chocolate.

ROD   After yoga class?

NINA   Yes. It's the first thing I do when I go home. First thing! Where's the chocolate? [laughs]

ROD   Don't put that in the book!

NINA   Why not? [laughs] Anyway, I feel good.

ROD   I've already said that I want to know what that means. Isn't there an emotional component to feeling good?

NINA   Yes, but what I'm trying to say is that the pleasurable sensations of doing yoga are like experiencing any other pleasure—like eating something that tastes good makes me feel good, right?

ROD   Yes, definitely. But for instance, sometimes you're at a really nice restaurant and you're eating really good food—I mean it definitely has an alchemical effect on your body and you're feeling good, but a lot of times it's fairly momentary. As soon as the good flavor in your mouth goes away the feeling is gone, but in yoga, when you come out of yoga class there is a lingering effect. It's not like you feel good only while you're in yoga class.

NINA   Okay. The metaphor I've been using for my relationship to yoga is that I'm attracted to it as if I was attracted to a person. People ask me, "Why do you do it?" For me what feels most truthful is to say that I was attracted to it, that I was drawn to it, like I am to some people.

ROD   Well, I think it's a good analogy. I don't think it's any more truthful than any other answers, but I think it's a good analogy in the sense that when you like someone else, usually it has a long-lasting feeling. You run up the stairs in front of you and you go home excited because you like somebody.

NINA   Yes, that's what I was getting at. But also, if you spend time with your friend—if you have a good time with your close friend or your lover—it is good and you feel good afterward.

ROD   Yes, maybe even for a long time! And then—what is feeling good again?

NINA   Oh. You don't think that feeling good is an emotion. You want me to say happy, contented, peaceful—

ROD   No, I think "good" is an emotion. I'm just trying to go a little further with what the elements of feeling good are, that's all. I'm just trying to get a little more specific here.

NINA   I guess a little more happy about being alive—just an appreciation of being alive and of feeling alive. More connected to life. I've definitely had some times in my life when being alive was really hard, really painful.

ROD   I think pretty much all of us on the face of the earth have faced that, and life is difficult sometimes. Really, really difficult, to the point of wondering if it's worth it.

NINA   Yes—I've definitely had a few moments where I felt like I was in such pain that I really just wanted it to stop.

ROD   This tape is about to stop. What a note to end on! Death. The possible alleviation of pain: death.

NINA   That's when I understood suicide for the first time. It wasn't wanting to be dead. It was wanting the pain to stop.

ROD   [whispering] The end of suffering. Maybe that's why we practice yoga. Maybe it even promises something that big.

NINA   [whispering] I don't believe it.

ROD   I don't really care what you believe. You should know that by now. Belief is nothing! Belief is nothing.

NINA   What do you care about what I *whatever?*

ROD   I believe I—

NINA   You—
        [tape ends]

A BREATH PRACTICE

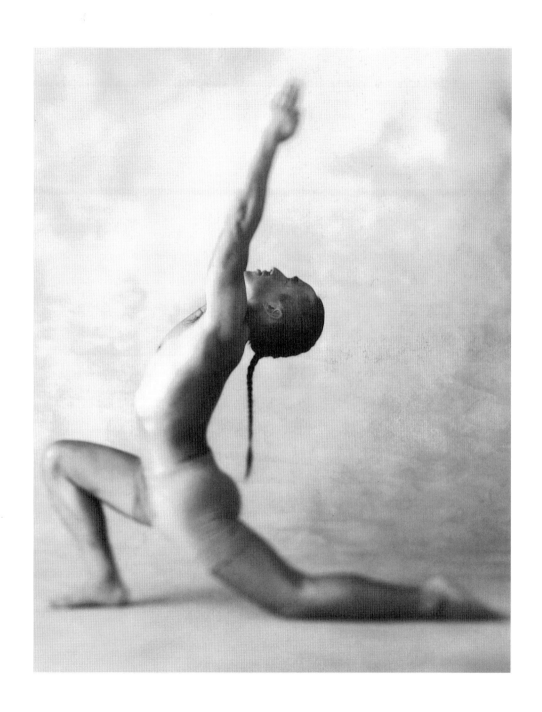

Considering the Practice

I celebrate myself, and sing myself,
And what I assume you shall assume,
For every atom belonging to me as good
belongs to you.

I loafe and invite my soul,
I lean and loafe at my ease observing a spear of summer
grass.
. . . .
Houses and rooms are full of perfumes, the shelves are
crowded with perfumes,
I breathe the fragrance myself and know it and like it,
The distillation would intoxicate me also, but I shall not
let it.

The atmosphere is not a perfume, it has no taste of the
distillation, it is odorless,
It is for my mouth forever, I am in love with it,
I will go to the bank by the wood and become
undisguised and naked,
I am mad for it to be in contact with me.

The smoke of my own breath,
Echoes, ripples, buzz'd whispers, love-root, silk-thread,
crotch and vine,
My respiration and inspiration, the beating of my heart,
the passing of blood and air through my lungs,
The sniff of green leaves and dry leaves, and of the shore
and dark-color'd sea-rocks, and of hay in the barn,
The sound of the belch'd words of my voice loos'd to the
eddies of the wind,
A few light kisses, a few embraces, a reaching around of
arms,
The play of shine and shade on the trees as the supple
boughs wag,
The delight alone or in the rush of the streets, or along
the fields and hill-sides,
The feeling of health, the full-noon trill, the song of me
rising from bed and meeting the sun.

— WALT WHITMAN,
FROM "SONG OF MYSELF"

Breathing. Your breath is what lets you move out of thought into feeling. A sensual and sensory process. Like smelling the morning smells from a distant village. So sip your breath. Take in its essence—that blend of subtle flavors that allows you to fall into that moment. And surrender into the trance of your breath.

Let your breath run your mind rather than your mind run your breath.

Breathing needs to be completely appropriate to what you are doing, fast or slow, shallow or deep. So observe your breath—don't judge, manipulate, or force it. And smell and taste it from the back of your mind.

Let the breath soak into your cells.

Surrendering. Just as you can open the doors and the windows in a summer house that has been closed up all winter but you cannot control the wind and the sun that begin to enter the rooms, you cannot control your breath. You must *allow* it. So surrender, open your doors and windows, and let your breath take over.

Dream your breath into your body.

Back Bends. Back bends open your chest and bring your attention to your breath. In back bends, your chest is expanded and your lungs are open. So why do you grip your breath? Can you learn to do these poses without gripping?

Passive Back Bend

Cobra

Locust

Bow Pose

Let it be the waves of your breaths that move you into the shape of these back bends. Feel how your breath runs over your internal landscapes.

Depth. Doing yoga deeply is not a matter of strength or flexibility or force but a matter of how *prana*—the wind of your body—is absorbed. Let your breath be the sponge that absorbs both your mind and your body.

Yoga poses that are absorbed, not performed.

1. Passive Back Bend

3 to 5 minutes

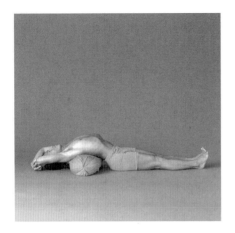

Instructions. Lie back against the blanket roll, with your shoulder blades resting on the top of the blanket roll and your head spilling backward. If your neck or head is uncomfortable in this position, you can place a pillow under your head.

Inhaling. Sigh. And sigh again. Notice the heaving of your chest. Then let all your inhalations be the kind that come after a sigh. *Natural, complete inhalations, short or long, deep or shallow.* Never force or hold your breath but simply receive your breath. Can you retain a deep receptivity in the center of your heart?

> *soft opening*
> *increased vulnerability*
> *increased exposure*

Exhaling. An orgasmic taste. Then the lingering aftertaste. So don't rush your exhalation. Let it linger, like the fog that rushes into San Francisco Bay through the Golden Gate but that never rushes back out. We watch it hover in a fine mist over the bay, gradually getting lighter and lighter as it slowly burns off in the summer sun.

Let your breath take over. And as a wave slowly retreats back into the sea, letting itself be absorbed by the sandy shore, let your lingering exhalation be absorbed into the tissues of your body.

One Thing. Your body is a room, and your ribs are venetian blinds hanging over the windows that you have just opened. And your breath is the sunshine and fresh air that are just beginning to stream in. Feel it. Observe it, but don't manipulate it. *The beginning of spring cleaning.*

2. Cobra

10 to 15 breaths
Repetitions: 1 to 3 times

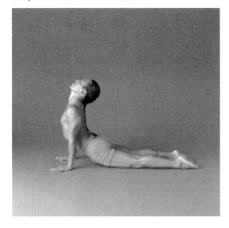

Instructions. Lead with your legs, not your head. Ground your legs, and keep your waist long—front, sides, and back—lifting more from your side body and chest. Then let your neck and head follow. Don't be afraid to move back and forth, side to side, to work out all the kinks. *A belly dance.*

One Thing. Rise naturally from a deep letting go, as the morning mist rises from the earth. And let it take *that long*—the natural rising—the undulation of the spine that peels back from the surface of the earth. Like an orange peel spraying its fragrance—a beautiful fragrance set free.

3. Locust

5 to 10 breaths
Repetitions: 1 to 3 times

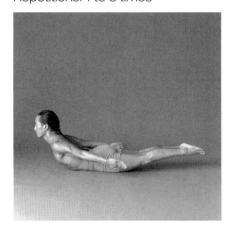

Instructions. Lengthen your legs, and draw them together. Then slowly move your chest and head forward and up as your legs move back and up. Work your back muscles strongly, but don't just contract your back—let it have an extended, broad feeling.

The evenness of the arc is what's important, not the height of it. Concentrate on contracting evenly from the soles of your feet to the crown of your head—equanimity in length, width, and depth, so that every fiber of your body is engaged.

Now immerse yourself in your undulating body as it rises and falls with your breath like the currents and swells of the sea. Feel the winds of your body—the way you live in your breath.

One Thing. Can you take on the shape and vibrational quality of a locust? And even if your breath is quick and shallow, taste your breath in the back of your mind. Try it with your eyes closed to be more aware of the fragrance of your breath, the aftertaste of your breath.

4. Bow Pose

5 to 10 breaths

Repetitions: 1 to 3 times

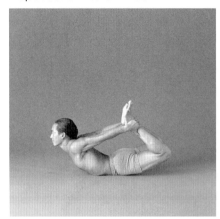

Instructions. As you hold your ankles, lift your legs. Feel your belly and pelvis narrow and hollow (don't let them be pushed into the ground by the lift of your legs). Lengthen your waist, move your chest forward, and let your head follow your chest. But always, always leave space for your breath. Let it flow into your body as if into a hollow reed or a flute, sounding and re-sounding.

> *legs strong*
> *spine long*
> *chest open*
> *arms drawn*

Moving Out. With a slow, smooth exhalation, lightly release back to the ground. Like a strong wind that stills for a moment.

One Thing. As you slowly rise into this back bend, let the pitch of your body rise but stay even (like the pitch rising on the string of a violin). Your breath will be shallower, but let it resonate deeply. Listen to the sound of your breath. Don't judge, manipulate, or force it. The pose tells you—if you allow it—how you should breathe.

5. Hero Pose
15 to 30 breaths

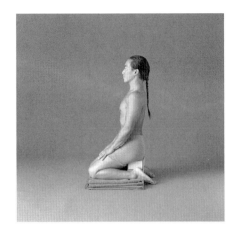

Instructions. Sit right between your feet, on a prop (a block or blanket) that is high enough so that you can exhale completely and so that the tops of your thighs feel like they are dropping toward the ground. Allow your thighs to drop completely as your pelvis begins to float. Let go of any gripping behind your forehead, your jaw, and your temples.

legs dropped
waist long
chest open
head balanced
exhalation complete

One Thing. Feel the tension of your legs dissipate. When our minds are full of desire or aversion, our legs naturally want to propel us toward our desires or away from our aversions. So our legs rarely rest. Let them rest now.

By resting your legs, you are giving your breath a reprieve. Like stopping to take in the view while hiking up a mountain. The fullness of the breath returns.

So take these moments. Let them be like clearing your palate with water before tasting a different wine.

6. Legs Up the Wall Pose
3 to 10 minutes

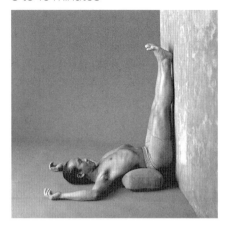

Instructions. Place your legs as close to a wall as possible with your sacrum resting on the ground and the backs of your thighs pressing against the wall. To open your chest, position a blanket so that the bottom tips of your shoulder blades hit the blanket's folded edge while your shoulders release to the floor.

Let your legs be a waterfall cascading into the pool of your belly. The blood now drains easily back into your torso. Your legs no longer have to work to return your blood to your heart. *Rest.*

One Thing. Cool lemonade with a sprig of mint on a hot summer afternoon. Cooling the mind. So drink it in. Breathe as if you are taking in the air after a fresh morning rain. Ethereal air. Where the condor soars.

And bring your attention to your breath. If your attention wanders, gently bring it back again. In this pose your breath tends to flow naturally. It is a good example of what your breath is like when not forced or blocked. A breath you can learn to bring into the rest of your life.

7. Reclined Cobbler's Pose
3 to 10 minutes

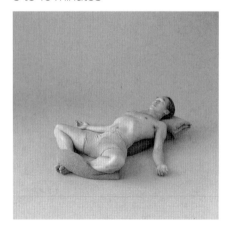

Instructions. With your head higher than your chest and your chest higher than your belly, bend your legs and let them drop open to the sides, with the soles of your feet together. Everything cascades down from your chest—belly, legs, pelvis—like a river spilling into the ocean.

> *legs fallen*
> *belly receptive*
> *chest full*
> *mind luminous*

If this irritates your inner thighs or pelvis, place a folded blanket under each knee.

One Thing. This pose invites your understanding of breathing into your groins. Providing a sense of security within vulnerability. The security from being so grounded, with open groins and legs, belly, and heart all exposed. A rocking rhythm. A cradling. The sound of your breath is the sound of water, water rushing down your body into the earth, chaotically, continually.

8. Relaxation Pose

5 to 10 minutes

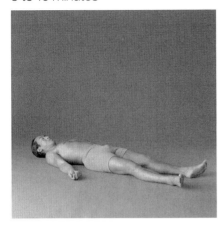

Instructions. Drop your boundaries. Let your bones feel heavy and your sense organs empty—the ethereal, vital life force pulsating, coursing through your veins and arteries. Feel the vitality of surrender.

The silence after music. A scintillating tone—ringing clear as a bell throughout your entire body—as your breath rises and falls.

> *legs below belly*
> *chest below head—*
> *mind descending to heart*
> *arms like folded wings*

One Thing. Listen to the sound of your breath moving through the universe of your inner body, finding no resistance. Can you let your breath become your consciousness, harmonizing with the sounds and rhythms of your surroundings?

An endless continuation of sound through space, sounding and resounding, like a conch shell horn.

9. Sitting Meditation

5 minutes or intuition

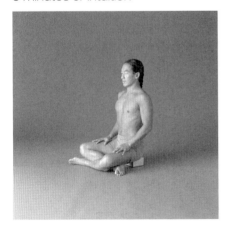

Sitting. Sit in a simple crossed-legged position. Continue to try to sit so that your body is completely responsive to your breath. Lifted, but not too lifted. So your breath resounds as movement in the skin of your body.

Meditating. Remember when you were a child and you stayed for so long in the pool that your teeth were chattering and your lips turned blue and your fingers and toes were "raisins"—and your mother kept calling you to come out, but you just kept putting it off—"just a couple more minutes, Mom, just a couple more minutes"—and when you finally did come out, and your mother wrapped you up in a warm, dry towel, you ran over to a patch of bare, baking-hot cement and plopped right onto it, belly down, so your shivering little body could absorb all of its heat?

As you sit, can you absorb the many layers of your breath the same way you once absorbed the heat of the pavement through your chest and your belly?

Reconsidering the Practice

When you get involved with and intrigued by the breath, it becomes interesting to watch it all day long. Can you become conscious, but not self-conscious, of your own and other people's breath? *Am I free with my breath?* (A free breath is not necessarily a slow, calm breath but rather a natural, appropriate breath. If you are upset or angry, your breath is not slow or calm, and you need not force it to be. Let it run freely.)

Are you talking to someone you're not comfortable with? Notice where your center is and how your breath is. Then see if you can recenter yourself and relax your breath. You don't have to hold a stressful internal pose.

You will still get angry, afraid, and worried, but can you be immediate about letting it go, like a small child, instead of carrying it with you through the entire day? Have you ever watched two small children coming to blows over a toy one moment and then playing happily side by side the next? Screams of frustration and bitter tears of anger only to be followed by contentment.

The practice is simply this: keep coming back to your breath during the day. Just take a moment. This will give your mind a steadiness and your breath a gracefulness. And before you go to sleep, spend a little time lying on your back in a comfortable position. Instead of thinking of what went wrong during the day or planning what to do the next day or counting sheep, pay attention to your breath.

There's so much to let go of, isn't there? Your nostalgia and your regrets. Your fantasies and your fears. What you think you *want* instead of what is happening right now. *Breathe.*

BREATHING

The first thing she does is look at the clock—eleven-thirty—damn, that means she slept about an hour and then woke up again, abruptly, for no reason—not a good sign—it's like that song by the Talking Heads—can't sleep my bed's on fire—don't touch me I'm a real live wire—and she was already stretched to her limit, with a full day at the office to get through tomorrow, David on a business trip, the nausea of her second pregnancy dragging her down, and a three-year-old to care for—that's what she worries about most, being a good mother—oh, God, all she wants, the only thing she really wants is to be the way she *used* to be, a woman who slept the whole night through and who could move through the world with an oblivious ease because of that (she has to admit, her twenties had been disappointing and even a little sad, but there had been one thing that she could count on: every night she would slide her naked body on top of David's and breathe in the warmth of his fragrance— whole wheat toast, ginger snaps, and fermented apples—and then when she was just on that blissful edge, he would nudge her gently and she would roll onto warm sheets, and morning sun coming in through a window would be the next thing she knew), and aching from the loss of that, she hears the sound of crying from another room, and then she panics, what can I possibly say to comfort my little girl, my little string bean, when I can't even figure out how to get through the night myself? but when she carries her daughter into her own bed and lies down beside her, her child relaxes back into sleep without a word, and she realizes that all the little girl needs is the scent of her mother and a warm, breathing body next to her, and suddenly it is the easiest thing in the world to do what is necessary, just live through the night one breath at a time, and that's all I'm going to say because even if I told you whether the woman soon fell into a deep, dreamless sleep or stayed awake until dawn, whether she went to work or spent the day in bed crying, or whether she lived sixty years with her husband, raising children and grandchildren, or fell in love with her drawing teacher at thirty-eight and ran off to Barcelona, her story will only end when she dies, and I much prefer to leave her just where she is, breathing.

—NINA ZOLOTOW

Breath Practice Summary

1. Passive Back Bend
3 to 5 minutes

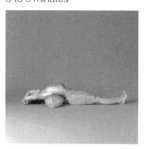

2. Cobra
10 to 15 breaths, 1 to 3 times

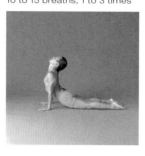

3. Locust
5 to 10 breaths, 1 to 3 times

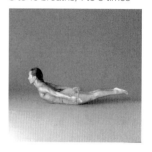

4. Bow Pose
5 to 10 breaths, 1 to 3 times

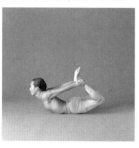

5. Hero Pose
15 to 30 breaths

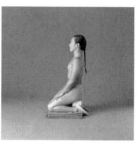

6. Legs Up the Wall Pose
3 to 10 minutes

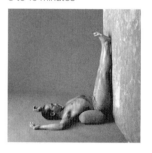

7. Reclined Cobbler's Pose
3 to 10 minutes

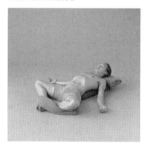

8. Relaxation Pose
5 to 10 minutes

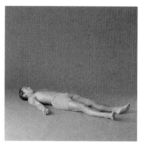

9. Sitting Meditation
5 minutes or intuition

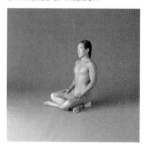

The End of Suffering

NINA   Actually, I don't believe yoga can end suffering, but I hope that it can help me cope with grief and pain so—so I don't become unhinged by it.

ROD   I think yoga *can* end suffering. I think that what it cannot end is pain, sadness, and difficulty. That's different from suffering.

NINA   Let's define *suffering*, then.

ROD   To me, suffering is what happens psychologically—it's more like how you attach to the feelings. What you do with the feelings is different from the feelings themselves.

NINA   Can you explain that in more concrete terms? You know how you were talking in class about the difference between reading something and feeling it in your body? And the difference between the way we just talk about things and then when we use a visceral metaphor—how it resounds in the body? If you only say these words *suffering* and *grief*, it's all just abstractions. You need vivid detail.

ROD   I agree. So here's a vivid detail. Let's say you have a physical pain. For instance, we can produce a physical pain in yoga and often we do. Maybe stretching your hamstrings is sort of painful, but if you watch the pain deeply, if you watch the sensation and deeply observe the sensation of your hamstring stretching, then actually you don't ever really identify it as *pain*. What I'm trying to say by this is that by going *into* the pain, in some sense, you realize that you don't actually have to *suffer* from the pain. For instance, take Stephen Hawkings. His body is mutilated and I'm sure he's in physical pain. But in some ways, it feels like his approach is simply "My body is still functioning well enough to maintain life, and I still have the ability to be in complete awe of the nature of the universe."

So what I'm saying is that you can have sadness and you can have pain, but it doesn't necessarily have to produce suffering. Suffering is what happens when, for instance, if you have a pain in your back, you say, "Oh, woe is me, I have a pain in my back. Oh, woe is me, I can't go swimming because I have a pain in my back. Oh, woe is me"—it's like this whole sort of self-wallowing. Instead, why can't you go ahead and feel what you feel instead of suffering from that? I mean literally be liberated by it.

NINA   So your child has just died—

ROD   You know, my good friend Ian, his baby was stillborn. And I lived with him after the baby died. In other words, I was his next-door neighbor the whole time. And you know what? He hated when people felt sorry for him because he said, "You guys don't understand the experience. I'm living this. You don't understand it. I'm not suffering from it—I'm living it." It was so powerful. So he didn't suffer from it, but people kept on trying to make him suffer. That was a whole different experience. People kept on wanting to feel sorry for him, and that was going to bring suffering, but being in it was not suffering. Being *in it* was the most difficult thing you could probably be in ever, but in some ways it was extraordinary because he was *forced* to follow it. You're in the moment-by-moment transition of the feeling as it changes shapes. And maybe you even have a happy moment—you might even have a happy moment in the midst of feeling deeply sad. You might have surprisingly sad moments at the weirdest times—maybe the feeling comes back. So it actually makes you *follow*.

So I think the grief is real, and I think, yes, the suffering is there from the grief. But I don't think it's necessary, though. I think a person can have grief without suffering, to actually feel the grief completely and not label it but keep feeling the movement of grief. I think that what happens is the suffering is actually when you identify with the grief and you start holding on to it instead of actually following moment by moment the ache in your heart.

NINA   This is interesting, but I'm confused. The ache in your heart—following it. That isn't like letting it go. It's following it. So suffering is caused by not letting yourself feel the grief?

ROD   Yes. It's falling *out of* feeling. A good example of what I'm trying to say is Emily Dickinson. She was very insecure and experienced depression and a lot of difficulties, but in some ways what she did as a poet was to keep on dropping so much into the feeling that she *was* the feeling. She *was* the difficulty, so that in some ways, I don't think she suffered from it.

So one can have difficulty, and one can experience that difficulty and even continue to follow the different shapes of that difficulty. And the more you *follow* it, the less you suffer from it. Because, for instance, let's say you're sad. Let's say you're feeling the different movements of your heart. It's getting more convulsive. Your breath is getting uneven, and so on. You're feeling a shape in your body, and if you keep feeling it, there's no room for suffering. You're ever present with the feeling.

NINA   That is something I definitely don't yet comprehend on a visceral level.

ROD   This is what Krishnamurti talked a lot about, and which I am really beginning to understand in my yoga practice. Let's say, if you saw a dog with three legs—

NINA   Right.

ROD   Does the dog look like it's suffering, necessarily?

NINA   No. That's actually a great metaphor because, just when you said, "if you saw a dog with three legs," I immediately remembered having understood that when looking at one. They just accommodate and they live.

ROD   That doesn't mean they're not in pain.

NINA   But they seem perfectly as happy as other dogs.

ROD   Yes, they don't say, "Oh, I have three legs and oh, woe is me." And this is what Krishnamurti was saying. He said, if you keep following just what you are and who you are, and you're following your life, are there any judgments or comparisons? You don't have any time to compare. If you don't have time to compare, you can't suffer.

NINA   Well, I'm not there yet.

ROD   Well, that's okay. I'm just saying that these are the things that are possible in yoga. And how is this possible in yoga? Yoga teaches you to continue to be present moment by moment by moment. How does it do that? First of all, it hones your concentration. It hones your concentration initially in your body sensations. So you're having these body sensations and you're taught to keep following them. Well, what's the sensation now? What's the sensation now? What's the sensation now? It's not like, oh, I'm going to compare this sensation with yesterday's sensation. No. What is the sensation now? Train your mind to be present now.

Then you even go to the breath, which is more subtle. It's training your mind to be focused on the subtle and keep bringing it back. Keep bringing it back and say: How does my breath feel? How does my breath feel? How does my breath feel? Then you're just following your breath. It starts becoming a motion picture instead of a freeze-frame photograph. For example, what happens when you go see a great film or listen to great music? Sometimes the concert ends and you realize that you've been present the whole time. You've been intrigued the whole time.

I remember when Donna left me for a while after ten years of marriage. And of course it was the saddest time in my life, but you know what? I was also really present. I was following moment by moment the movements of my sadness. Was I suffering? In some sense, no. I only suffered when I could no longer follow the movement. I actually suffered when I no longer followed the sadness.

NINA   Give me an example, because that gets too abstract for me. Give me an example of a moment when you did suffer or when you didn't suffer—

ROD   For instance, when she first left, I was sitting on the couch looking at the mantel—at our fireplace—and I remember how vividly I was seeing the mantel, how in some sense my whole world had been deconstructed and I was left bare with the present moment. And it was like, yes, I'm feeling heavy and sad, but at the same time I'm feeling what's going on. And actually, the times that I would suffer the most were the times when I wouldn't see what was going on. I couldn't actually see anything in front of me. I was so—it wasn't—

NINA   What was happening when you were suffering? What were you thinking?

ROD   I was intellectually thinking about it more. I wasn't actually feeling my heart anymore. I was actually sort of—my mind was suffering. I was no longer even feeling.

NINA   What was your mind saying to you?

ROD   It was going through the future or it was going through the past.

NINA   So was it saying, "How am I going to live without her?" Stuff like that?

ROD   Yes. Instead of being right where I was, it was in some fictitious place—for example, if only I could have her back, instead of *she's not here right now.* She's not here right now and this is how I'm feeling. Instead, I was thinking, oh, if I could only have her back, I would feel this other way.

NINA   Right.

ROD   That's suffering.

NINA   Right. That's why I'm trying to get you to be specific.

ROD   I know—well, I'm pissed off.

NINA   This is interesting.

ROD   I like it.

NINA   What? You like being pissed off?

ROD   No, this is just—like you say, recently I've been teaching with passion. This is just passion coming out.

NINA   Well, I was pushing you. You're always pushing me when we're talking.

ROD   Well, good. I don't mind being pushed. No, I'm happy to be pushed because I want to explain these things because they're actually getting more and more clear to me, and I realize some of this philosophy is not clear to other people.

NINA   You know why? Because everyone sticks to the abstractions. It's like reading books about philosophy. They just go on and on—

ROD   I agree with you on some level, but on another level I believe that people are actually not willing to follow their own thoughts. This is what Krishna-murti was talking about. Not only can they not follow the present moment of a feeling, but they also can't follow their own thoughts. That's what I'm trying to do in the yoga practice: I'm trying to get both myself and others not only to follow physical sensations but also to follow thoughts. *Follow the thought.* Be tenacious with it. That's hatha yoga.

NINA Well, that's really interesting to me because that's what I do when I'm writing my stories. I sit there and when an idea comes up, it's like I tie myself to these wild horses and just let them drag me off wherever they want to go. And I always thought—you're going to laugh—that it was the opposite of yoga because in yoga you need to let go, right? You need to *not* be carried away, right? And in my writing, I do what I call "going for broke."

ROD That *is* letting go. That's the *real* letting go because you're letting your mind fly into where it's flying. Most people don't understand what letting go means—they think it's some New Age—

NINA Well, actually I think I do understand it in my writing, but I don't think I understand it in the rest of my life or in my body or in my emotional life.

ROD Letting go is, in some sense, letting whatever's arising, arise. That actually *is* letting go. You're letting go of the restrictions, of the binding, of the habitual fear.

NINA Most of my life I've been a rather reserved person, but there have also been times when I did go over some kind of edge—when I did go all the way with everything, and—well, you know about my breakdown. So it's not always okay for me—believe me—to go for broke.

ROD Well—come on—that's the issue we all face. That comes into yoga in every way: physically, mentally, emotionally. It's like accepting what arises and accepting the movement of where it's going and not necessarily saying, "Oh, well, then, I guess we're all going to become serial killers because that's what it's going to lead to." That's what some religions actually say about yoga. In fact, in Georgia, I read an article in a newspaper that quoted the Catholic Church as saying, "Yoga is dangerous because it clears the mind and leaves way for the devil." I mean, get *that*.

NINA Yes.

ROD It clears the mind and leaves way for the devil. That's amazing to me, but in some sense, I realize people actually think that. We've actually been trained *not* to think. It's like in yoga class, people think it's about stilling the mind. It's not about stilling the mind. It's about *following* the mind. It's really about deeply following something. What we're doing is we're disciplining the mind so that it can continue to follow the present moment, watching things arise as they arise. Watching thoughts arise as they arise and actually being cognizant of life as it's arising. To really be in it—otherwise you're not living a life. You're living an illusion of a life. You're actually disassociated from what's really going on.

And this is what Krishnamurti says. He says most people are living in images. In other words, you see a tree, and if you relate it to something you've seen before—you relate it to the symbol "tree"—then you actually never see what's in front of you. You never touch the bark. You never smell the leaves. You never sit under its shade. It's like we've gone so far now that . . . Here's a good example: We took a videotape of our kids and our kids were right there. And it's almost like we put on the video and the video was more real than looking at our kids. We were all excited at looking at the video of our kids. It's like we'd rather look at the video of our kids than our kids.

NINA   You want to know something? I don't have any videos of my kids. I feel a little bad about it, but I can't bring myself to do it for exactly that reason. So I have none, and a lot of people will think I'm a bad mother, right? No videos of my children.

ROD   The Chinese wouldn't allow themselves to get photographed because they thought it stole the spirit.

NINA   Yes.

ROD   And what I'm beginning to see is that—

NINA   Actually, I'm starting to feel really guilty—

ROD   They're going to hate you.

A RESISTANCE PRACTICE

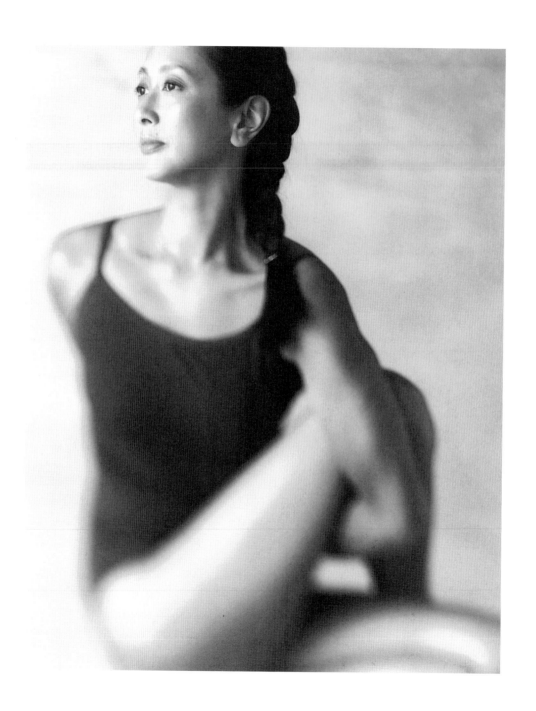

Considering the Practice

THE BEAVER POOL
IN DECEMBER

The brook is still open
where the water falls,
but over the deeper pools
clear ice forms; over the dark
shapes of stones, a rotting log,
and amber leaves that clattered down
after the first heavy frost.

Though I wait in the cold
until dusk, and though a sudden
bubble of air rises under the ice,
I see not a single animal.

The beavers thrive somewhere
else, eating the bark of hoarded
saplings. How they struggled
to pull the long branches
over the stiffening bank . . .

but now they pass without
effort, all through the chilly
water; moving like thoughts
in an unconflicted mind.

— JANE KENYON

Resistance. Life can be hard. And we are all prisoners sometimes, trapped in our cars in traffic jams, on crowded buses, or in windowless offices, or stuck in difficult relationships with family members, coworkers, or neighbors, or faced with disease, difficulty, and death. Resistance arises. *How do you meet it?*

Difficulty. Some yoga poses are difficult. You will find some poses uncomfortable and some painful. And there may be some you have a resistance to even approaching. *Which poses are difficult for you and why?*

Restriction. You have limits. Everyone does. Your hamstrings, hips, or shoulders are tight. Your arms, back, stomach muscles, or legs are weak. But this is your body—the body you have now, the body you have today. *Can you let go of your resistance while acknowledging your restriction?*

Breathing. Remember when you were a kid and you would walk along railroad tracks or a narrow ledge, and you would be totally engaged with the effort of just staying on track? And if you fell off, you would simply get back on and keep on going? *When you meet difficulty in a yoga pose, can you stay on the track of your breath?*
    Breathe. Inhaling. The sea sponge filling back up. Exhaling. Releasing your breath to its complete minimum.

Twisting Poses. In the twisting poses, you encounter the cycle of resistance.

> *resistance*
>   *pause*
>   *breath*
>   *space*
>   *movement*
>   *resistance*

Reclined Thigh-Over-Thigh Twist

Bharadvaja's Pose

Seated Crossed-Legged Twist

Marichi's Pose 3

Easy Lord of the Fishes Pose

1. Cobbler's Forward Bend

15 to 30 breaths

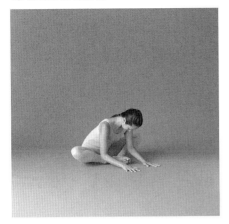

Instructions. Keep your focus on the release in your hip sockets, especially as you come to the point of resistance. Feel your liquid pelvis pouring over your thighs—whether or not you get much movement. Breathe in your belly, trying not to lock up. Cascade your spine forward from the hinging of your pelvis into the gradual release of your neck and head.

Release from the wideness of your back muscles, broadening from your spine, like grass in a field lying down in the wind.

Move more on your exhalation. Let your mind be soft, listening to your breath. Easing forward. Slow-motion falling.

> *drop your legs*
> *raise your chest*
> *spill your pelvis*
> *cascade your spine*

One Thing. Feel the resistance, then breathe into the resistance. Comprehend patience, like water smoothing a rock in a riverbed. The rock is your resistance. The water is your breath.

2. Wide-Angle Forward Bend

15 to 30 breaths

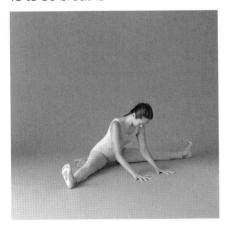

Instructions. Keep your legs and feet as strong as you can—in the direction of your heel bones, in the direction of your toes, in the direction of the balls of your feet—while allowing the core of your body to be as soft as possible.

> *broad feet*
> *strong, grounded legs*
> *falling torso*

One Thing. Be patient. Wait until you feel a sense of space. Then move on your exhalation. Wait again. Observe again. Move again.

3. Reclined Leg Stretch

15 to 30 breaths per side

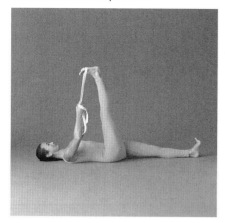

Instructions. Allow yourself to feel the contact of your body with the ground. Pull the strap lightly to bring your raised leg toward your chest, and feel the resistance in the back of your hamstring and your calf. Then, again, the grounding of your bottom leg. Then, again, the resistance of your raised leg.

> *wave of resistance after*
> *wave of resistance after*
> *wave of resistance after . . .*

One Thing. Feel the resistance. Find the space. Like water running downstream over all obstacles, sticks and leaves, stones and fallen trees. Let your exhalation draw the contour of your spine.

4. Reclined Thigh-Over-Thigh Twist

10 to 15 breaths per side

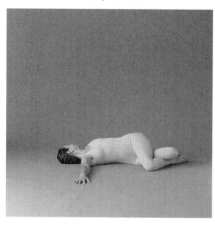

Instructions. Keep your feet and legs awake. Let the weight of your legs, chest, and arms create the action of the twist. Breathe in your belly and your back.

One Thing. How much and how far to let go? Observation and feedback tell you. Like a house cat stalking a bird.

> *pause*
> *observe*
> *wait*
> *space*
> *move*

Let intuition rise up to tell you how much to surrender.

5. Bharadvaja's Pose
10 to 15 breaths per side

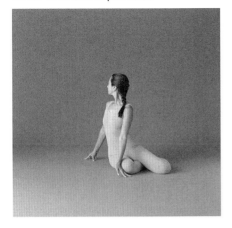

Instructions. Initiate the twist from your pelvis as it moves over your legs. Let your breath fall all the way down into the base of your pelvis and into your groins. Can you maintain a sense of evenness and spaciousness? Can you turn without getting kinked up, spiraling with ease and evenness?

One Thing. A cleansing action. Compression and release. Exhalation and inhalation. The sky dense with clouds, heavy and oppressive. Then it rains. Then a sky so clear you can see the outline of a mountain the way you've never seen it before.

6. Seated Crossed-Legged Twist
10 to 15 breaths per side

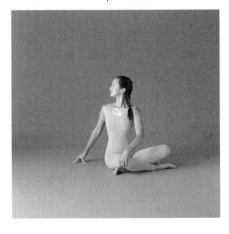

Instructions. With your right shin in front of the left, your pelvis and spine rise from your grounded legs. Exhale and turn to your right.

Since this pose is easy, it may be difficult for you to see the resistance. Therefore be more attentive to understand centering and balance. This is not about twisting more but about the coordination of your breath and how your breath wants to move in the twist.

> *exhale and turn*
> *inhale and back off*
> *observe and align—*
> *exhale and turn*
> *inhale and back off*
> *observe and align—*
> *exhale and turn . . .*

One Thing. When you are bored—or when things are really easy—see if you can hone your attention more. In some sense, this is one of the most challenging poses. But like feeling easy with a person—someone you're really close to and feel accepted by—if you stop paying close attention to him, it can lead to unexpected struggle.

7. Marichi's Pose 3

10 to 15 breaths per side

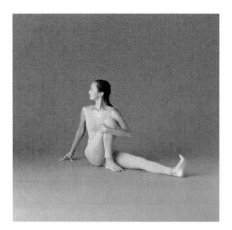

Instructions. In using your arms to help you move into the twist, can you feel them as an expression of your heart and lungs rather than the determination of your mind?

Keep a sense of space and ease of breath. Don't be aggressive or forceful. And don't lead with your head. Make sure you can exhale completely and freely.

> *root your leg*
> *lift your chest*
> *empty your belly*
> *spiral the twist*

One Thing. Move from the openness of your heart. Especially in this twist, there should be a real focus on your heart and lungs, on your lifted, open chest. Remember having a balsa wood airplane when you were a kid, and how you would wind up the rubber band that was attached to the propeller, watching closely as the rubber band coiled up tighter and tighter until it finally started to knot, and how you would then gently toss that airplane into the air and it would fly?

8. Easy Lord of the Fishes Pose

10 to 15 breaths per side

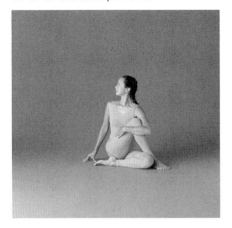

Instructions. The genesis of this twist is your hips—can you move into the resistance of the outer hip of your upper leg? Let go of the resistance at the base, at the foundation.

A spiral with no beginning and no ending.

> *legs rooting*
> *pelvis spinning*
> *chest continuing*
> *head completing—*
> *legs rooting,*
> *pelvis spinning*
> *chest continuing*
> *head completing—*
> *legs rooting . . .*

One Thing. Always from the earth up, not from the head down. Initiate the twist from your relationship with the ground, not from the desire of your mind. *A whale breaching—launching its body into the air and then arcing as it twists back into the sea.*

9. Cobra

10 to 15 breaths
Repetitions: 1 to 3 times

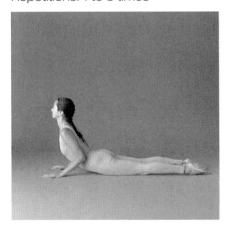

Instructions. Bring your attention to evenness—maintain both broadness and elongation. Move slowly as you are coming up, and try to maintain a symmetry between the left and right sides of your body.

Are you wondering why this pose comes after a series of twists? Sometimes twists broaden the muscles around your sacrum and spine, opening the back asymmetrically. You may be vulnerable. Cobra creates a new symmetry, revitalizing your back and allowing you to knit your body together, to rebuild your foundation, to reestablish the support of your spine.

One Thing. Feel the beautiful arc of your spine, from the arches of your feet to the crown of your head. A line like the crescent shape of a new moon. A melodious spine, like an Indian raga weaving a melody over a rhythm.

10. Supported Bridge Pose
15 to 30 breaths

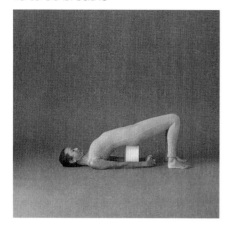

Instructions. Use a prop that is low enough so you are comfortable but high enough so your chest is open. Your shoulders and head should be on the same surface. However, if this irritates your neck, you can place a blanket under your shoulders and release your head softly back from them.

Now look at the openness of your chest. This pose is partly inverted, so the blood from your legs and pelvis easily returns to your heart. Bring an ease and expansiveness to your heart and lungs as you turn inward.

Your breath returns to a natural pattern. Your legs might be hard to root. Maintain some focus on keeping your legs strong and active—you can even tie your thighs together if you wish.

One Thing. You are meeting the resistance of being vulnerable and at the same time having to look at yourself in that vulnerability. Your chest is open, your pelvis is exposed, your arms and legs are helpless. Can you simply rest into that resistance?

11. Relaxation Pose
5 to 10 minutes

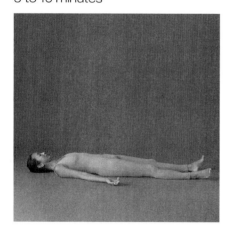

Instructions. Lie down. Do nothing for once.

Relaxation Pose is always important, but it is especially important after twists. However, it might not be so easy to do this pose now, or rather, it might be especially difficult. The twists might leave you feeling agitated. But can you simply let Relaxation Pose open the dam to flood the plains?

> *lie with the binding of your body—*
> *the tangle of human complexity—*
> *exhale and let it unravel*

One Thing. We're partly defined by our resistance. What we're up against. What we don't like. What we don't believe. But what would happen if you were completely neutral?

12. Sitting Meditation

5 minutes or intuition

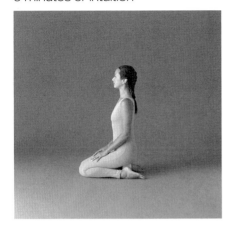

Sitting. Sit in Hero Pose (appropriate for meeting resistance, don't you think?). But sit on a prop that is high enough so you are comfortable.

Hero Pose—at this point in your life—may feel like a terribly unnatural pose. But if you visit countries where people do not sit on chairs, you will find that adults have retained their childhood ability to fold their legs deeply in this position. You can let your legs return to their natural suppleness by practicing this pose. With time, this pose will help your legs lose some of the stiff resistance in your hip, knee, and ankle joints, returning them to their natural freedom, both in sitting and in walking. (How wonderful walking with freedom can feel, how utterly, utterly wonderful.)

(If you want to meditate longer than five minutes, come out of Hero Pose and assume your traditional sitting position.)

Meditating. The galaxy of your own being. Notice all that arises and falls in your body—thoughts, physical sensations, feelings . . .

> *spiraling*
> > *chaotically*

Give and take. An unwinding and a winding. A winding and an unwinding. Release from the resistance. A moment of fresh air for the prisoner.

Reconsidering the Practice

As resistance comes up during the day, what is your relationship to it? Do you:

> *avoid it?*
> *fight against it?*
> *cower and subjugate yourself to it?*

Can you have a little fun with it? Like a dog who brings a stick to his master—he wants to give the stick up so his master will throw it for him, but he enjoys a little bit of struggle first—the master trying to pull the stick out of his mouth—*grrr*—before he is ready to let it go.

Resistance is an intriguing part of our lives—doing things that are hard for us, doing things we are afraid of. It's our work *and* our play. Like the dance of two people getting to know each other, two people in love before they've admitted it to each other. Cary Grant and Rosalind Russell. Katharine Hepburn and Spencer Tracy. Beatrice and Benedick in *Much Ado About Nothing.*

So when you find a yoga pose that's really difficult for you, it's a good one to take into your practice—in a curious, interested way—to help you understand more about your body and your life. Because when there is resistance in a yoga pose, it occurs because you have a mental concept of what you'd like the pose to be that is in conflict with what your body is capable of doing in the moment. But can you simply back up your expectations and be involved with what is happening right now? Isn't that enough?

WHAT IS ENOUGH?

I believe life is worth living—although once I considered overdosing, not because I wanted to die but because I was in such pain—would the scorching of my heart ever end, would it ever, ever end?—that I just wanted to stop feeling, but the thought of my children prevented me from opening the cabinet and uncapping those orange plastic bottles because I understood that I could endure anything for them—on the other hand, the thought of suicide has consoled me periodically—once while I was swamped with love for my own husband, I was throttled by a terrible fear—how could I live without him?—and then I suddenly understood that I didn't have to live without him, that I had a choice, and I felt a great sense of relief; but all in all, I'm a very curious person, and I think that's what will always keep me going: how will the book or movie end? what will happen to me tomorrow? who will I love next? and if I do ever write another story—of course I will, won't I?—what will it be? and that woman sitting next to me, why does she always carry a glass jar of tea with her wherever she goes? and what kind of tea is in it? and what does it taste like? (she tells me that her jar of tea is the thing she loves most in the world, that she even took it with her when she went to Israel, and she doesn't know what she loves more, the tea or the jar, and then she lets me hold the jar—it really does feel lovely, the heat from the tea radiating out through the smooth, curved glass into my hands—and she pours a little of the tea—branch tea—into my cup, so I get to taste the intense earthiness of it, and I tell her that I am fascinated by her fascination with her tea jar), and isn't that enough?

—NINA ZOLOTOW

Resistance Practice Summary

1. Cobbler's Forward Bend
15 to 30 breaths

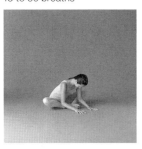

2. Wide-Angle Forward Bend
15 to 30 breaths

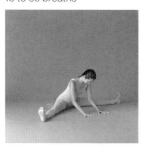

3. Reclined Leg Stretch
15 to 30 breaths per side

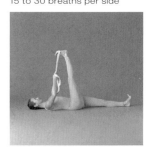

4. Reclined Thigh-Over-Thigh Twist
10 to 15 breaths per side

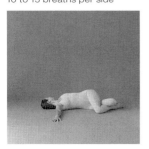

5. Bharadvaja's Pose
10 to 15 breaths per side

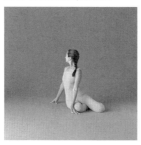

6. Seated Crossed-Legged Twist
10 to 15 breaths per side

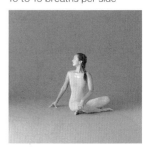

7. Marichi's Pose 3
10 to 15 breaths per side

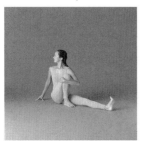

8. Easy Lord of the Fishes Pose
10 to 15 breaths per side

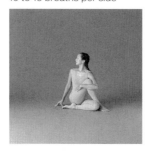

9. Cobra
10 to 15 breaths, 1 to 3 times

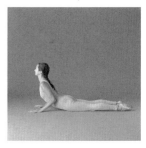

10. Supported Bridge Pose
15 to 30 breaths

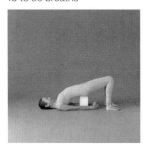

11. Relaxation Pose
5 to 10 minutes

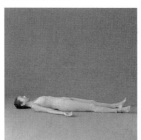

12. Sitting Meditation
5 minutes or intuition

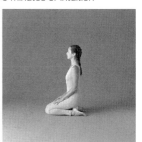

Meeting Resistance

ROD   What do you do, or what happens inside of you, when you have resistance? What's going on? Do you want to continue to meet resistance the way you always meet it? Or are you interested in inquiring about what the nature of resistance is in yourself? For instance, what do you have aversions to in your life? Do you—maybe—dislike your next-door neighbor? Is there resistance to being friendly with your next-door neighbor? And what are you going to do about that? That comes up in the yoga practice. There are certain postures that you like and don't like. There are certain resistances that come up in the yoga practice, and who are you when the resistance is there?

NINA   For me—today—that back bend over the block was very difficult. Why is it so much worse doing it over a block than over a bolster? But anyway, while I was doing it—because it was so painful and uncomfortable—I was definitely turning all that stuff over in my mind.

ROD   What you're saying is a really interesting thing. Here you have a yoga posture or something in yoga that's bringing up resistance. You basically just don't want to do it, and yet at the same time there's some impulse to think that it may be just exactly the thing that you need to do.

NINA   Well, I figured that out fast.

ROD   Okay, so what is it in our human psyche that may know that something we're resistant to may actually be something that we need to go into? I think it's really a natural seeking of balance. If you always do what you want to do and what you like, I think what that does is really bring you out of balance as a human being. We sometimes need to go toward the things we don't like and where we have resistance. That's the nature of a very important philosophical concept in yoga: to come to a place where you're not always trying to push away the things you don't like or attract the things you like. Because otherwise the world becomes this really small place based on your dislikes and likes, and there's no way you can actually enjoy a lot of things life has to offer.

NINA   That makes me think of Dorothy Allison, the author of *Bastard out of Carolina*. Have you read that novel? It's an extraordinary book because it's so brave, so authentic, and so powerful. It's about an abused girl and her family. But anyway, I read somewhere that what Dorothy Allison said about writing was "Go where the fear is." And that's one of my things that I tell myself to do in my writing. I remember last year I confessed to you that I have this list of things I'm too afraid to write about—that I keep this list and that I go back to it again and again. Because I realized that this exploration is where the most interesting and powerful things come up.

ROD   Exactly. That's exactly how it is in yoga. The places where you have the most resistance are actually the places that are going to be the areas of the greatest liberation. I mean I look at it this way: when you have issues with something—when you have difficulties with something—that means you're not at peace with whatever that is. And I think that a really important concept in yoga is that one can come to a deep sense of peace. Even though you may want to change something, there's still a deep acceptance of what is. I think that's a really basic thing. To have a deep understanding and acceptance of what is in this moment, in this present moment. That doesn't mean you're not going to put out elements of effort to try to change things for the future, but at the same time you're really observing what is. But if you have a lot of resistance, then basically your observation is nonexistent. The greatest learning comes with confronting the things that we have issues with.

NINA   Well, I gave my example—that I had a list of things I was too afraid to write about and I would write about them, or some of them. But do you have any examples of your own?

ROD   What am I scared of? Maybe I'm scared of not spending enough time with my children and doing what my father did—not really being around or being present with his children and then expecting later on in life to have some type of relationship that he doesn't have. I mean it just hasn't evolved. So I don't want to repeat that. But when I'm trying to be different from my dad, I encounter some resistance because I think that's the way I grew up, that's the way I've been imprinted, in some sense, so maybe I have a tendency to father the same way he fathered me.

And I think that yoga gives me the ability to meet that resistance. I mean it's really helped me, because for twenty years in yoga I've done poses that I didn't really want to do, like Hero Pose, which embarrassed me because I had to sit so high up, on so many props, but after a while I mastered them to a certain extent. Maybe I didn't master them as far as being able to do them like some picture in a book, but I mastered them in the sense that I didn't have an aversion to them anymore. I actually enjoyed being in their presence, in the presence of the poses that I used to hate.

And so these tendencies in my life to maybe be absent from my children—there's a strong pull toward that, and so there's a resistance to meet. And I feel like because I've met resistance, real physical resistance—there are things that churn in your belly, things that fluctuate in your heart, things that flip in your mind—and you can deal with that stuff. You can sit with that stuff. You can actually *be* in the difficulty and say, "I can be in this feeling where maybe my gut's going to throw up or my heart is going to palpitate, and I'm going to feel like I'm having some psychological fit or something, but I can stick with it, stay with it, meet that resistance." Usually when you do that, there's a major liberation that takes place. You can change philosophically, or you can change in actuality and manifest the changes you want to manifest.

NINA   That's really interesting for me to hear you say that. I have some strong reactions to it because for myself—observing your life—it disturbs me how often you're gone from your family. I know that this is because it's one of the issues I have with my husband—although he's never done it to the extent you do—but there were times in the past when he was away too much. Like the time I had a miscarriage, and he was in England for two weeks, so I had to go through the whole thing alone.

ROD   I mean, you want to know a men's issue in this country—we've talked about a lot of women's issues—but a big men's issue in this country is, how many people in our generation had fathers who were home? Most of the people I talk to—most of the friends I talk to—their fathers either weren't physically there or they weren't psychologically there. And personally, my dad was always on missions. He was flying missions. He was very social. And the beautiful thing is his family still came first in a lot of ways. I mean his really deep concern was his family. I have that myself. But you know, these are the things I'm struggling with, and these are the things yoga is helping me with by allowing me to observe my tendencies and clearing the way for new actions.

NINA   I'm glad you told me that.

ROD   There's another thing I think yoga really does: yoga is a way of taking responsibility for yourself in a lot of ways. You're responsible for keeping yourself healthy, and you're responsible for actually coming to the rest of the world in a more neutral state so you're a little more observant—

NINA   Not so quick to make a judgment—

ROD   I think you're a little less full of yourself, in some sense. It's a way of beginning to rid yourself of a lot of personal biases and ridiculous conclusions. I think that's a lot of the reason I practice yoga.

NINA   How does it do that?

ROD   It does that because the physical postures get you out of your physical habits, and it does that because your physical habits are a very specific vocabulary. You might say, Rodney Yee has a Rodney Yee walk, and Rodney Yee has a Rodney Yee way of talking. So people have their way of walking, their way of talking, their way of posturing in the world, and their philosophy in the world—their thoughts, the way they interpret things, their perception of the world. By doing postures, by breathing differently, by taking some time to create different shapes with your body, by thinking about different philosophical things, you get to a different perspective. You get to *feel* a different perspective in your body. You get to breathe a different way.

   That's a profound thing, to breathe a different way than you involuntarily do. It changes the body. It changes the mind. It changes your capability of seeing beyond what you've defined, of what your habit has defined as your reality. That's profound. Did you know that I can actually imitate other people? My body can actually get into different shapes.

NINA   Somebody was suggesting that you do that today—it came up in class.

ROD   I did—I imitated a bunch of people at the swimming pool, and they just loved it. They loved it because imitation doesn't just come with making the same physical movements, it comes with actually *understanding* different feelings, different shapes. That's what architecture's about, in some sense. If you go into a certain room where there's not much space, it creates a certain feeling compared with a place that's too big, like an airplane hangar. And then maybe you have something in between, like a cathedral that uplifts you in some inexplicable way. There is the architecture of the body. And your body taking different architectural shapes creates different feelings. It's not really much of a mystery.

People think, oh, it hasn't been proven by science yet. What do you mean, it hasn't been proven? How long have you been in your body? I go outside on a beautiful blue day and it has a certain effect on me and on my mood. I go out on a rainy, cold, blustery winter afternoon and it has an atmosphere. People talk about atmosphere all the time. I go into a house, it has a certain atmosphere; I go into a restaurant, it has a certain atmosphere. In fact, I go to that restaurant *for* the atmosphere because I'm in the mood maybe for a romantic atmosphere, or I'm in the mood for watching a sports game at a sports bar. Or I'm in the mood for being in a casino with a bunch of smokers and drinkers. Or I'm in the mood for being at my parents' house and feeling nostalgic. You know, there are different atmospheres! So I don't understand what's so mysterious about it—you create different shapes with your body and it creates different emotions!

NINA   Why are you so angry right now?

ROD   Because people think that it's some unproven thing! It's so simple. But people basically keep refusing to acknowledge it. Or maybe they just haven't even comprehended it.

NINA   Is it people? You haven't gotten any acknowledgment from me that—

ROD   From you? No, you're just one of many. Look at all the scientists who are running around dismissing yoga as some useless New Age fad because it hasn't been proved according to their methodology—

NINA   But why do you care what they think?

ROD   Why do I care what they think?

NINA   Yeah, why do you care what they think?

ROD   Because they have power.

NINA   What are they doing to you? Are they stopping you?

ROD   No, they just ridicule it. So I'm ridiculing them.

NINA   You're not ridiculing them, you're pissed off.

ROD   Well, yeah, I'm pissed off for being ridiculed. Is that such a big mystery? If someone ridicules you, doesn't it make you mad?

NINA   There's an area of resistance, I guess.

ROD   What bothers me bothers me.

NINA   That's what is interesting. That's what we're talking about.

ROD   Yes, but maybe "Why?" is not the question.

NINA   When you're looking at resistance, what is the question?

ROD   Maybe it's just *feel* the resistance.

NINA   Well, by asking "Why?" I'm just exploring it with you, right?

ROD   Yes, but in some ways it intellectualizes the resistance. It doesn't need to be intellectualized. It can be, and that's one way of looking at it, but—

NINA   So I can sit with you while you do it, so I can sit with your anger toward scientists and feel it with you. [laughs]

ROD   It doesn't need to be looked at with words, necessarily.

NINA   Well, that's the way I look at things, right?

ROD   Well, maybe not. I mean you're doing yoga and meditation, and that's another way to look at resistance. Meditation is a silent way of looking at resistance; it's not necessarily silent inside, but basically you're sitting with the resistance. You're not running away from it—you're sitting with it, you're stewing in it, you're fidgeting with it, but basically you're trying to follow the resistance. And I think that's very interesting!

You don't have to have a conversation with someone about the resistance. You might have your own little conversation inside your head about it, like, oh gosh, there I go again, I'm thinking about what I did yesterday, and I'm supposed to be just sitting here and watching my breath, oh, and now I'm thinking about that again, and why was that so important? . . . You know, you have your own little conversations in your head, but after a while in meditation you are bringing yourself back to now. And if you feel resistance, *feel* the resistance. It doesn't mean you have to figure it out, it doesn't mean you have to go anywhere with it, it doesn't mean you have to solve it—it might get worse, it might get better. You just don't know sometimes. Things arise. Resistances arise. And it's not necessarily something that you have to figure out. But definitely, if the resistance is arising inside you, you have really no choice but to be with it, in some sense, until it resolves or dissolves in its own right. And sometimes you have nothing to do with it resolving or dissolving. But to live it, to be in it, is actually a profound thing.

NINA   This ties nicely into the section in our book on breath observation.

ROD   Yes. Not only am I moving more toward meditation in my own practice, but also I've done *pranayama* [breath absorption] for fifteen years, and I love *pranayama*. I go to a place in my psyche and in my body that I'm not really allowed to go any other time during the day. And I mean that not just as a personal thing but as a societal thing. People don't allow you to sit and watch your breath. You have to do that on your own time. I can't tell you how wonderful it is to be that intimate with your breath and to be that intimate with your mind, to just be there, watching your mind move.

   And maybe that's what you love as a writer. In some sense, you're really with your own mind. That's why I think you called your domain *wandering-mind*, because you're with the wanderings of your mind. For the most part, when at any other job do you get to actually do that? You're supposed to be producing. That's why my friend Ian, the classical musician, sometimes doesn't want to play concerts. He doesn't want to have to *produce* music. He wants to *be* with the music. You want to *be* with your mind, as a writer. I want to *be* with my breath, as a yogi. I want to watch *it* and watch it so deeply that I *am* it. I *am* my breath. I *am* my mind. I'm not trying to do something with my mind. I'm not trying to produce something with my breath. I'm not trying to produce something with these postures or with this body. I'm not trying to get healthy. I'm not trying to get unhealthy. I'm not *trying* to do something with this. I'm doing it because I love to do it and I am doing it. Everybody pushes you in this life. "Why are you doing that? What are you doing that *for*? What's that going to lead to?" Well, it's all leading to death—so get it straight. You're going to die, okay?

A RELAXATION PRACTICE

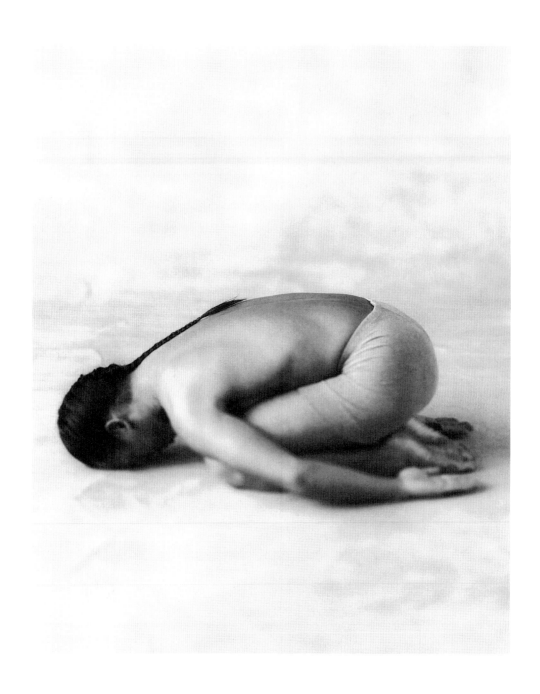

Considering the Practice

Napped half the day;
no one
punished me!

— I S S A

Turning Inward. In a relaxation practice, you don't need to hold yourself up any-more, not with your muscles and not with your determination. In quiet, supported poses, you can completely let go. Then you are free to observe the movement of—

your breath—
your thoughts—
the beat of your heart

Restoration. There is a restorative quality to the conscious rest you gain from a re-laxation practice that no amount of sleep can bring you. Because by asking your mind to dwell on the subtle movements of your body and your breath, you can access the potency of the present moment.

Resistance. Sometimes lying around and relaxing is difficult. You may find it easier to do an active workout—exerting yourself and sweating. So for some people a re-laxation practice can cause a different kind of resistance, such as boredom, agita-tion, or restlessness. But if this kind of resistance arises, simply observe it.

And often an itch will arise, physical, mental, or emotional. If possible, don't scratch it—breathe life into it. As you give the itch attention by breathing life force into it, you will observe its natural life cycle of—

rising
climaxing
descending
releasing

You don't need to *try* to rest. In this practice, simply noticing how you are *is* resting.

Forward Bends. By folding your body over itself, you are physically turning your senses inward and cooling and calming both your nervous system and your mind.

Crossed-Legged Forward Bend
One-Legged Forward Bend
Seated Forward Bend
Wide-Angle Forward Bend
Child's Pose

Supported Poses. Supported poses allow you to take different shapes with your body—bending or twisting or raising your legs over your head—without exertion. So just relax. Relax, breath, and feel.

Restorative Twist
Reclined Cobbler's Pose
Legs Up the Wall Pose

Warmth. A relaxation practice can cool you down. So do whatever is necessary to stay warm. However, if you become cold or uncomfortable during this practice, try to let go of it—see if you can deal with it by simply relaxing internally.

1. One-Legged Forward Bend with Chair

15 to 25 breaths per side
Repetitions: 1 to 2 times (right and left, then right and left again)

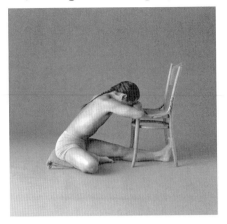

Instructions. As you come into the pose, extend your spine and draw the life force up through it as your torso grows upward and then rests forward. *Effort and surrender.* Ground and align both your bent and straight legs, and keep your feet awake and in constant responsiveness to their relationship with the legs.

One Thing. Can you relinquish the physical and mental effort that you use for being in the world?

Begin the journey inward. And savor that beginning. Like those wonderful lighthearted Friday afternoons when you leave work before the start of a two-week vacation. Let go of the external pulling. Feel free to wander around inside your own body as if you were simply puttering around the house on an unexpected day off.

2. Seated Forward Bend with Chair

15 to 25 breaths

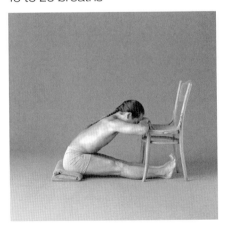

Instructions. Sit with a blanket under your sitting bones. Let this pose be about clarity. Clear the energy in your legs and draw it into the extension of your spine. Don't overstretch a single part of your body. Keep your legs working evenly and feeding evenly into your torso. Search your body for symmetry and equanimity.

One Thing. Can you surrender in the midst of resistance without collapsing? Meet resistance with steadiness and attention and not by giving in to pain or discomfort. Feel an attentive willingness to subjugate yourself—not a giving up but a moving inward with receptivity. Create a clarity through the physical posture that allows your breath to circulate freely throughout your body. *A turtle pulling its limbs inward and resting under the dome of its shell.*

3. Wide-Angle Forward Bend with Bolster

15 to 25 breaths

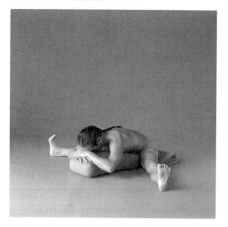

Instructions. Sit on a prop that is high enough so your pelvis can spill forward. Then rest your head and arms on a prop that is high enough for you to rest on easily (a bolster, a stack of folded blankets, or even the seat of a chair, as in the previous pose). Actively root your legs, drawing energy up through your spine—the circulation of your breath is inside that activity. *Resistance.* The backs and insides of your legs will speak to you loudly. It's obvious that you are stretching them. But can you still feel a sense of your legs gathering energy from the ground?

More than any other seated pose, this one gives you a feeling of having a broad, wide foundation. The strength and grounding of your legs, along with the relaxation and ease of your torso, allow your foundation to become more profound and assured.

One Thing. Exhilarating expansion with a quiet core, like a hawk spreading its wings over a huge landscape. Let your mental body be as wide as it can be. And allow the horizontal lines of your body to bring contentment and tranquillity.

4. Crossed-Legged Forward Bend with Bolster

1 to 3 minutes

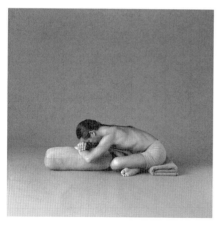

Instructions. Rest the weight of your torso and head on the bolster, and let the fibers of your neck unravel, turning your senses inward. Allow your central nervous system to melt downward toward the cauldron of your pelvis.

Let your legs fall into the ground, feeling filaments of light streaming from the arches of your feet into the base of your spine, through the conduits of your legs. As your spine is lightly arced from your tailbone to the prostration of your forehead, feel the humility of this pose.

One Thing. Feel completely supported, and drop still further into your internal space. Continue to contact the earth through your crossed legs. Retain the heat in your body as stones at night retain heat from a burning desert sun.

5. Supported Child's Pose

3 to 5 minutes

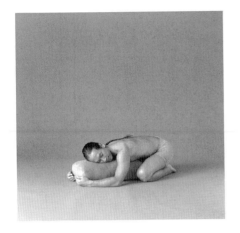

Instructions. Your entire torso should be supported, from your pelvis to your head. Let your spine be like the back of a tortoise, gently arching from your tailbone to your head.

The entire front of your body—the vulnerable part—is now supported and protected. Like a warm and solid embrace. And your back muscles lengthen and spread. Let the contact of your front body with the blankets or bolster help you understand the tension you hold in your body. See it and then let it go.

If you've turned your head to one side, be sure to turn it to the other side when you are halfway through your time in this pose.

One Thing. Like an afternoon nap so deep that you drool on your pillow. . . . And deep sighs.

6. Restorative Twist

2 to 3 minutes per side

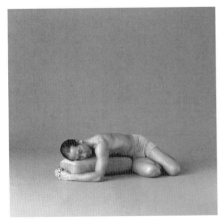

Instructions. As you lie down, unravel all your skin so it's not pinched or caught. Try to lengthen your bottom waist, and turn your head whichever way is the most comfortable.

Now feel your breath move into your groins, lower back, and sacrum—the center of your back body. Inhale and uncoil. Exhale and coil.

> *breathing*
> *pulsating*
> *resting*
> *dreaming*

One Thing. As the tension of the twist unwinds, let yourself know the safety of the container in which you lie. Like a small child who needs to be in its mother's arms before it can talk to a stranger. Allow the twist to give you a tactile knowledge of the resistance of your back. *Relaxation within restriction.* Within a given amount of space, you have an infinite playground for your breath and inner movement.

7. Reclined Cobbler's Pose

3 to 10 minutes

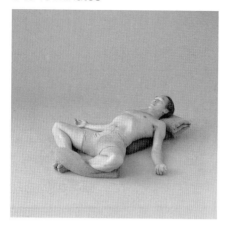

Instructions. Consciously allow your front body to drop more and more toward your back body. Feel your belly draining down into your legs as your heart expands.

What a vulnerable position. Your legs and belly are open—your arms are flung away from your chest. So it takes diligence for you to stay with the vulnerability. But once you do, the effect is quite resounding. *The boundless space into which you can fall.*

One Thing. Can you begin to unravel some of the mysteries of deeper relaxation? *"What is it?" you ask yourself. "What am I letting myself fall into?"* Savor the unknown and the unfamiliar.

8. Legs Up the Wall Pose

3 to 10 minutes

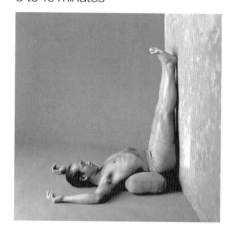

Instructions. Keep some activity in your legs as they press against the wall. Feel the weight of your legs falling down into your hip joints and the blood of your legs returning so easily to your heart. Feel the vulnerability of your chest in a back bend along with the turning inward of your neck and head in a forward bend. *The deep comfort of heavy wool blankets on a cold winter night.*

One Thing. Inverted comfort. This pose turns you upside down—giving you a complete change of orientation—but it also brings security. You have more contact with the ground—and the wall—than you do in Relaxation Pose, and this tactile sense of familiarity allows you to relax even as you are inverted. Let your breath begin to sink fully into its exhalation. *Feel the vulnerability of your heart.*

9. Relaxation Pose with Chair

3 to 10 minutes

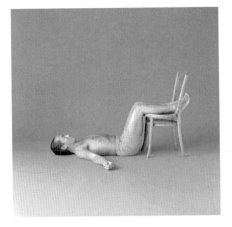

Instructions. With your calves on the chair, your lower back will be flatter and your sacrum will rest more easily on the ground. Surrender the weight of your legs to the seat of the chair. Your calf muscles are some of the most active muscles in your body. Soften them now, and realize that you can let go of their never-ending conversation with balance.

One Thing. As your back body widens and is fully supported by the earth, melt your front body downward into that support— your exhalation becoming like mist hovering above tall grasses, illuminated by the morning light angling through the trees. *Your mind cradled by the movement of your breath.*

10. Sitting Meditation

5 minutes or intuition

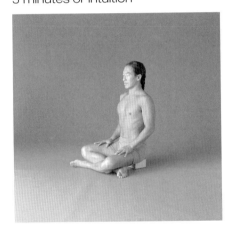

Sitting. Sit on a folded blanket or block in a simple crossed-legged position. Your legs and sitting bones provide the foundation for this pose. Press your sacrum toward the front of your body, elongating your side waist up into your spacious, airy chest, and press your shoulder blades into your back to give your chest extra lightness. Align your head with subtlety over your heart and pelvis in a continual, delicate balance.

As your mind resides toward the back of your skull, move your breath into your back body like a cloud moving onto a mountain, bringing moisture to the moss and lichen on the mountainside.

Meditating. Let your mind find its seat and begin to slow down, as if you were in the presence of giant coastal redwoods with their cathedral height and serenity. (California redwood trees are among the oldest living things on the earth—some live to be over one thousand years old. And throughout the year, they are both nourished and protected by the blankets of cool, white fog that drift into the coastal valleys from over the Pacific Ocean.)

Reconsidering the Practice

Let's face it—we live in a society that does not value relaxation. It's something we're supposed to do for two or three weeks every August. And the rest of the year, we're working in the office, and putting away the groceries, and folding the laundry, and repairing the roof, and weeding the garden, and baking brownies for the PTA bake sale, and shopping for clothes at the mall, and getting signatures on a petition, and driving the kids to soccer games, and exercising at the gym, and anything we do that doesn't produce results is "wasting time." But really, is there anything in your life that could not be done better and more fully through relaxation?

Because relaxation means doing something 100 percent, without worrying about the fruits of your action. And nonattachment to the outcome of your actions allows you to be fully present in the moment of action, the present moment. The more fully you can be engaged with your mind, body, and breath in this moment, the more you will be alive—

> *to feel*
> *to think*
> *to move*

Think of a paramedic: If he panics, he can't see what needs to be done. But if he can be present with all his faculties—his sense organs, his breath, and his mind—he is more capable of living that moment and responding appropriately.

But it's as if we've become so blasted with stimulation from the outside (just consider TV, which is supposed to be so relaxing—all those loud noises and jarring images bombarding you) that we're used to running at a certain RPM and don't even know how to turn the engine off. So when you finally allow yourself to slow down, it may be an unfamiliar feeling. *Zoning in, not zoning out.* And your mind will certainly wander. To the past and the future. To your nostalgia and your regrets, to your longings and your worries. But interruptions don't matter. When your mind wanders from the present moment—from your body and your breath—simply call it back. That mindfulness alone will bring relaxation and restoration.

WINTER

In their garden there was always a wild profusion of tomatoes ripening on the vine, and leafy basil, arugula, and lettuce, and glossy purple eggplants, and red and yellow peppers, and zucchini with its long, bright blossoms, and there was always lunch at the wooden table on hot summer afternoons, with plates of pasta and bread and olives and salads with herbs, and many bottles of red wine that made you feel warm and drowsy, while bees hummed and the sprawling marjoram, thyme, and rosemary gave off their pungent fragrances, and at the end of the meal, always, inexplicably, there were fresh black figs that they picked themselves from the tree at the garden's center, an eighteen-foot fig tree, for how was it possible—this was not Tuscany but Ithaca—Ithaca, New York, a rough-hewn landscape of deep rocky gorges and bitter icy winters, and I finally had to ask him—my neighbor—how did that beautiful tree live through the year, how did it endure the harshness of a New York winter and not only survive until spring but continue producing that miraculous fruit, year after year, and he told me that it was quite simple, really, that every fall, after the tree lost all its leaves, he would sever the tree's roots on one side only and, on the tree's other side, he would dig a trench, and then he would just lay down that flexible trunk and limbs, lay them down in the earth and gently cover them with soil, and there the fig tree would rest, warm and protected, until spring came, when he could remove its protective covering and stand the tree up once again to greet the sun; and now in this long gray season of darkness and cold and grief (do I have to tell you over what? for isn't it always the same—the loss of a lover, the death of a child, or the incomprehensible cruelty of one human being to another?), as I gaze out of my window at the empty space where the fig tree will stand again next spring, I think, yes, lay me down like that, lay me down like the fig tree that sleeps in the earth, and let my body rest easily on the ground—my roots connecting me to some warm immutable center— luxuriating in the heart of winter.

—NINA ZOLOTOW

Relaxation Practice Summary

1. One-Legged Forward Bend with Chair
15 to 25 breaths per side, 1 to 2 times

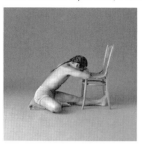

2. Seated Forward Bend with Chair
15 to 25 breaths

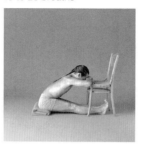

3. Wide-Angle Forward Bend with Bolster
15 to 25 breaths

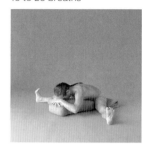

4. Crossed-Legged Forward Bend with Bolster
1 to 3 minutes

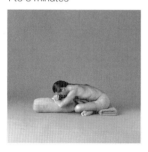

5. Supported Child's Pose
3 to 5 minutes

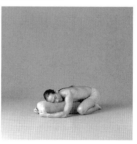

6. Restorative Twist
2 to 3 minutes per side

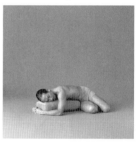

7. Reclined Cobbler's Pose
3 to 10 minutes

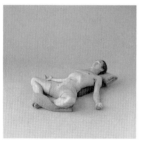

8. Legs Up the Wall Pose
3 to 10 minutes

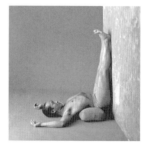

9. Relaxation Pose with Chair
3 to 10 minutes

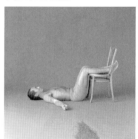

10. Sitting Meditation
5 minutes or intuition

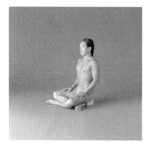

The Yoga Mind Game

NINA   You recently said, "I really hate the way yoga's being talked about these days." What did you mean by that?

ROD   I hate the way yoga's being talked about because, in some ways, as we talk about yoga we talk about it as some ultrapositive experience, as if it were still involved in the duality of the positive and the negative, as if it's going to create some great positive thing in your life and it's going to eradicate the negative things in your life. I think it really does aid people in getting what they want, but I think it also can make one pass over some things that are really important to just be *with*. Yoga is a way to be with whatever is, so it's not a matter of getting better or changing things from what they are, so much as sitting with *what is*. But I feel like it's talked about as some healing or transformative art, as if we're supposed to beam ourselves up into some heavenly place or as if we're here in an earthly hell from which we're supposed to levitate ourselves.

NINA   Yes. It's like so many of the books out there on the market now on "self-improvement." They're all about getting happier, wealthier, more successful, healthier, and I think that in a lot of people's minds yoga fits into that category. Is that what you're talking about?

ROD   Yes. In my mind, it's not much different from . . . Here you go—when I was in Hong Kong my cousin was really into this guy who has a company that teaches you how to be successful by using mantras, an ancient form of concentration. For example, you might make a mantra of "I will be wealthy. I will be successful," and say that to yourself a hundred times a day. And it's having some success—I don't doubt that it can work—but the problem is that people start using these practices as a means to *achieve*. They think that they're supposed to achieve something with the practice, and that, to me, is the very downfall of understanding. It's actually a deep misunderstanding of the practice. And yet, you might say, why do you do it then? Aren't you trying to get somewhere, aren't you trying to do something with it? But like I've said to you before, no, I just love the practice for what it is.

NINA   One of the things that I'm curious about is the kind of expectations you see in people when they come to yoga class.

ROD   Well, I don't even think it's just what they come to class with. I think it's what they walk around with every moment of their lives, and that is thinking that they're supposed to be someone that they're not. And so they come into the classroom with exactly what they're walking around with every second in their heads: I want to improve myself. I have to get better. I have to get thinner. I have to be smarter. I have to be wealthier. I have to be a better person. I have to do this. I have to do that.

It's just an endless rat race that produces exactly what they don't want, which is a feeling of inadequacy, because basically they're never what they want to be. And so you're left with one constant feeling of dissatisfaction as a human being, and that is ultimately suffering moment by moment by moment.

NINA   My son had this great teacher in fifth grade, and she usually gave him very original and stimulating assignments. However, at the beginning of the new year, she gave him the following assignment: "Please write down fifty new year's resolutions." And Quinn was just miserable. He did not want to do this assignment because he did not want to sit and think about fifty things about himself that needed improving. And the more I talked to him about it, the more I realized he was absolutely right. And he got very upset about it because he's a very conscientious student and he didn't like the idea of not turning in his homework. So I called his teacher at home (she was great about letting students call her anytime they wanted to) and talked to her about the problem, and I asked if Quinn could, instead of doing the assignment, write her a letter saying why he felt this was a bad assignment. So he wrote her that letter, and we also talked for a long time about why people even make resolutions. Because the kinds of things people resolve every year just become burdens on them the rest of the year. Why don't we make some resolutions that we can keep?

ROD   Like what?

NINA   Well, Quinn's final resolution was just this: pet more dogs. And that whole year we actively pursued keeping that resolution while we were out on our walks. We walked up to people and asked, "Can we pet your dog?" and they would say yes, and we would kneel down on the sidewalk and pet their dog. We petted so many more dogs that year than we had ever done before.

ROD   [laughs] Well, maybe, if it becomes a game like that, then it's sort of interesting and fun. But most of us are pretty damned ugly, very stupidly serious about our new year's resolutions because deep down inside, we want to do these things, and we feel very incapable because we can't achieve them, and yet even the ones we do achieve, they seem, after a very short while, worthless.

So it's a mind game, and it's like you see it over and over again in yourself as you're practicing yoga. You see the whole mind game reoccur. And you see it as a yoga teacher because people come in with all kinds of different goals and ambitions. In fact, I was just interviewed recently for a public TV show, and one of the main questions was: should people come in with goals and ambitions? And I said that's the very thing that's going to keep you from actually being involved in yoga—coming in with all kinds of lofty ideas and ambitions and goals. It's like, can't you just come in and be with yourself, and be with your body and look at your foot? And the teacher might say, "Ground your inner heel because your inner heel's not grounded." But it doesn't matter necessarily to even ground the inner heel or not to ground the inner heel. It's really more a matter of just, *can you see your foot?* There are all sort of tricks to say, well, let's just be here looking at our bodies, being in our bodies, feeling our bodies, listening to our minds, listening to our breath. And if you don't, that's fine, too. It's more like feeling who you are and what you are, and it's not so much an achieving of anything.

NINA   Yesterday I heard all kinds of stories about teachers taking people and forcing their bodies into certain poses, you know, pushing them really strongly, as if it was really important for them to be in that pose no matter what, even if it might injure them.

ROD   You have to watch out. I went through this as a yoga teacher, too. As a teacher you want to get people deeper into the pose because the people themselves will feel like they actually achieved something and then they'll give you the credit for helping them achieve something. So it's like this constant candy for everybody. Let's say you came in and you wanted to do a handstand, and let's say I was able to get you up in a handstand in one class. Then all of a sudden you're really happy because you achieved handstand. And then you give me some gratification and you bow down to me because I helped you get into handstand, and it feeds everybody's ego. But after a while you do that enough times and you start to realize, wow, my ego's big and now it's small again, now it's big again, now it's small again, and after a while it just seems like that would lose its attraction. But we seem to be able to do a lifetime of that.

NINA   [laughs] Some strange addiction.

ROD   Yes. So I think as a yoga teacher, it's a fine line of having some of the skills to help people with their bodies and their minds and yet at the same time not becoming involved in that.

NINA   What do you mean, "not becoming involved in that"? Do you mean not having your ego attached to whether they achieve what you think they should achieve or not? Is that what you mean?

ROD   Yes. It's more like, they're here, and you have these arbitrary goals, but you have to realize that they're arbitrary, that they're not really what the practice is about. The importance of the practice is not to get gratified all of a sudden because you achieved these goals. It's more like the goals are just ways to pay attention, and the goals themselves are actually not the important things. It's the ability to pay attention and *sustain* your attention that we're honing.

NINA   During some of our earlier discussions, you talked about why you did yoga in the beginning. You said it brought you hope, but you said also that you don't practice for that reason now. Why do you practice now?

ROD   I'm not sure if I said this before, but in my early twenties I became—unbeknownst to myself—fairly depressed. I didn't have the outward forms of it because I was always very gregarious and had a lot of fun with people. But I think I was actually depressed. Because I had a lot of ideas about the world, that it could be peaceful and jovial, and people could be in community, and people would share their belongings. And I really didn't understand why that wasn't happening. I didn't understand why communism didn't work and why people wouldn't, basically, let everybody have the same amount of everything, and why we couldn't all live in some fantasy harmony and help support each other, both emotionally and physically, and welcome people into our house and our home. I really was wondering that as a ninth grader. I was like, what's the problem here?

And I learned also of my own difficulties with being that way, that I wasn't so free to give and love and be in community, that I had my own selfish difficulties and egoism, and so I started realizing the difficulty of the world. And I think that was ultimately depressing compared to the lofty ideology of my younger years. And my college years were even more training in getting further and further away from any sense of communion or harmony—in fact, I felt like my college years were about creating more division, more judgment, and more harshness.

And so when I first started doing yoga, at least I felt on some level the joining of my philosophical beliefs and my physical reality. For example, there was my ability to believe in vegetarianism and to actually become a vegetarian, and an ability to be in much less internal conflict with all of the voices screaming inside of me, and an ability to make peace with people who in the past I had had extreme conflict with. So yoga gave me some form of hope in the sense of my being able to be a little bit more what I thought I should be.

But as the years have gone on, I feel like the practice is more about *not believing,* about *not* having hope, about *not* thinking that there's supposed to be anything but what is. The more I sit and listen, the more I feel like I'm in touch with the nature of things as they are instead of just having hopes for how I would like things to be. There's amazing joy, extreme sadness, the dullness of the mundane—the entire scope of human existence. It's all going to come through you.

A MOVEMENT PRACTICE

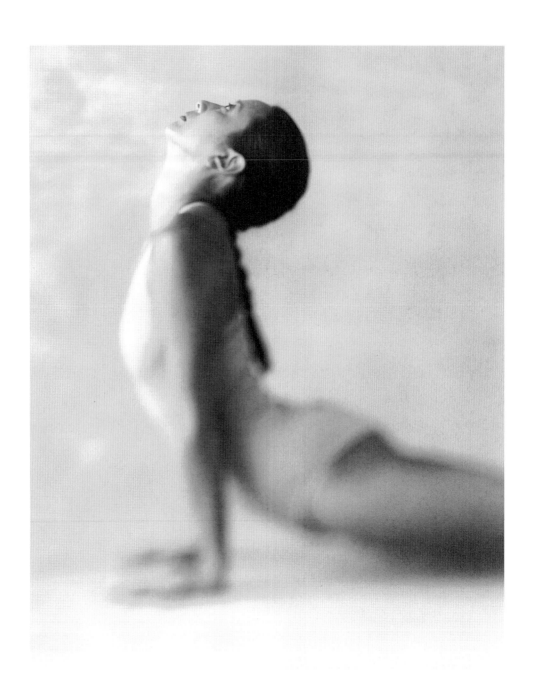

Considering the Practice

It would be more decorous not to live. To live is not decorous,
Says he who after many years
Returned to the city of his youth. There was no one left
Of those who once walked these streets.
And now they had nothing, except his eyes.
Stumbling, he walked and looked, instead of them,
On the light they had loved, on the lilacs again in bloom.
His legs were, after all, more perfect
Than nonexistent legs. His lungs breathed in air
As is usual with the living. His heart was beating,
Surprising him with its beating, in his body
Their blood flowed, his arteries fed them with oxygen.
He felt, inside, their livers, spleens, intestines.
Masculinity and femininity, elapsed, met in him
And every shame, every grief, every love.
If ever we accede to enlightenment,
He thought, it is in one compassionate moment
When what separated them from me vanishes
And a shower of drops from a bunch of lilacs
Pours on my face, and hers, and his, at the same time.

— CZESLAW MILOSZ

Movement. You are never completely still. And as you sensitize yourself to your inner forces, you can let your outer movements be initiated by your core inner movements.

moment by movement by moment

Posing and Reposing. While you are posing, you are observing. And from that observation, you intuit a movement. Then you repose. These movements can bring you awareness of your habits and help dissolve them, layer after layer.

Sun Salutations. A Sun Salutation is a series of poses that you link together with movement and breath. This teaches you that the movement between poses is as essential as the movement within poses.

> Mountain Pose
>
> Volcano Pose
>
> Standing Forward Bend
>
> Extended Standing Forward Bend
>
> Lunge
>
> Downward-Facing Dog
>
> Plank Pose or Push-up Pose
>
> Upward-Facing Dog
>
> Powerful Pose

Riding the Breath. The flow and rhythm of a movement practice allow you to observe the ebb and flow of your breath and help you become intuitive about how to ride it.

> *letting it rise*
> *letting it suspend*
> *letting it fall*

Part 1: New Poses

The previous practices in this book introduced some of the poses in the traditional Sun Salutation, including Mountain Pose, Standing Forward Bend, and Downward-Facing Dog. This section introduces the five new poses you need to learn before doing your first full Sun Salutation. Part 2 of this practice tells you how to link all these poses together using movement and breath.

By the way, there's no One Thing for the poses introduced in this practice, because for each Sun Salutation that you practice, we will give you qualities to practice within the salutation.

1. Volcano Pose

15 to 25 breaths

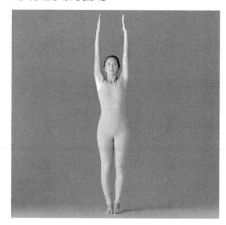

Instructions. Start in Mountain Pose. From the foundation of your legs, as you inhale, slowly raise your arms out to the side. Yawn your arms. Stretch. Challenge the elasticity of your dormant muscles. Pull the breath up your body. Then reach your arms above as if you were just getting out of bed in the morning—your energy surging through your body and up and out your hands.

> *thrusting, pushing arms*
>> *sharp, extending legs*
>>> *lifted, expanding chest*
>>>> *stretched, elongating waist*

2. Extended Standing Forward Bends

5 to 10 breaths

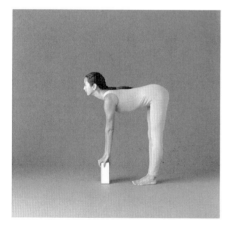

Instructions: To enter this pose, extend your spine forward on your inhalation. Be willing to come up as high as you need to get a full extension of your spine. And place your hands appropriately—on blocks, on your thighs or anywhere down your legs, or fingertips on the ground—to encourage the extension of your spine. Keep your legs strong and your back body broad, with a continuous movement into extension to the very core of your heart.

> *earth-driven legs*
>> *broad-flaring back*
>>> *upward-growing spine*

3. Lunge

5 to 10 breaths per side

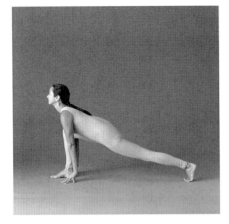

Instructions: To enter this pose, first bend both your legs and then reach one leg back into the lunge. Keep your pelvis square while you extend your back leg strongly, like a runner pushing against a starting block, as your front leg reaches for its maximum stride (up to but no more than 90 degrees). *Two legs pulsing in opposition.*

Can you bring the same energetic opening of your chest to this pose that you did to the previous pose, Extended Standing Forward Bend?

> *branched legs*
> *squared hips*
> *expanded chest*

4. Plank Pose or Push-up Pose

1 to 5 breaths

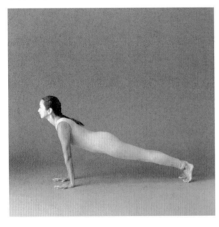

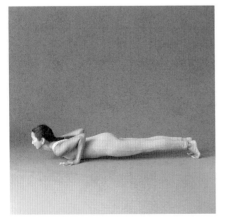

Instructions. To enter this pose, start from Lunge. Then step your front foot back to meet the back foot. Find the straight line from your heels through to your chest as you gaze forward from fully extended arms.

Bend your arms only as much as you can while still keeping your chest open and lifted. Keep your elbows close to your sides, your hands as even on the ground as possible, and your fingers spinning outward as your arms gather into the forward movement of your chest.

Fuse your two strong legs together into a single powerful channel of energy while keeping your feet very alive and feeding into the leg. *The potent tail of a dragon.* Allow that energy to move up through the core of your heart to the crown of your head.

> *legs in line with each other*
> *pelvis in line with your legs*
> *core of your heart in line with your pelvis*

5. Upward-Facing Dog
3 to 5 breaths

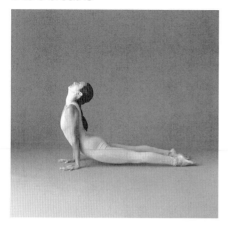

Instructions: To enter this pose, start from Plank Pose (above). Then move onto the tops of your feet—one foot at a time—and deepen your sacrum as you lift your chest.

Maintain the strength of your legs, from feet to hips, as you lift your thighs mightily from the floor. Keep your arms strong, too, like trunks of trees supporting the canopy of your chest. Allow your spine to receive the energy from both your legs and arms as you bend into the shape of a crescent moon, your head and neck residing gently at the top.

> *arches lifted*
> *thighs lifted*
> *sacrum deepened*
> *belly hollowed*
> *chest resurrected*
> *spine arched*

6. Powerful Pose
5 to 10 breaths

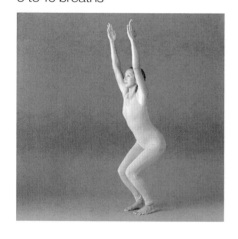

Instructions: To enter this pose, start from Standing Forward Bend. Then bend your legs up to 90 degrees while maintaining the press of your heels into the ground. Next, bring your body toward vertical, with your arms over your head, and gaze forward.

Try to keep your shins moving forward over vibrant feet, the tops of your thighs pressing downward to the ground through your heels, your pelvis lifting off the coiled springs of your legs, and your arms bursting up from the clear channel of your torso. Your pelvis is the underground water, and your arms shoot upward from that source like the geyser.

> *taloned feet*
> *coiled legs*
> *surging pelvis*
> *sparking arms*

Part 2: Sun Salutations

First Salutation

Let your first Sun Salutation be a *gentle* practice. How can you explore gentleness in these poses? By coordinating your movements with your breath. By going only as deep in the poses as you can while allowing your breath to flow easily.

1. Stand in Mountain Pose, noticing your breath.

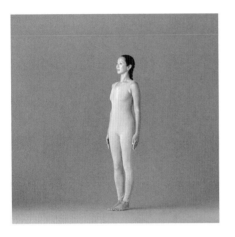

2. Inhale and raise your arms above your head into Volcano Pose.

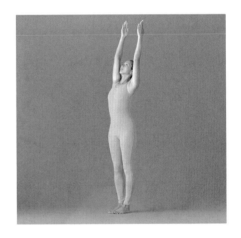

3. Exhale and swan-dive forward into Standing Forward Bend.

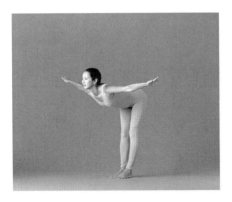

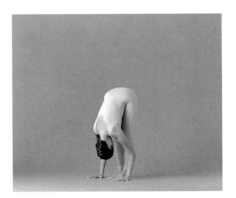

4. Inhale and lift into Extended Standing Forward Bend.

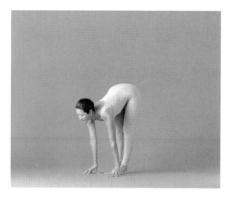

5. Exhale and bend your knees, then reach your right leg back into Lunge.

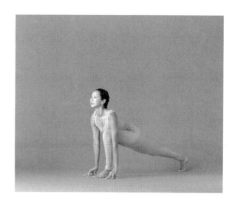

6. Inhale, extend and expand Lunge.

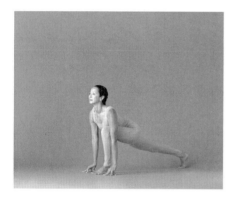

7. Exhale and move into Plank Pose or Push-up Pose.

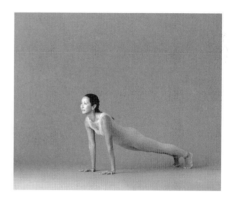

8. Inhale and arch into Upward-Facing Dog.

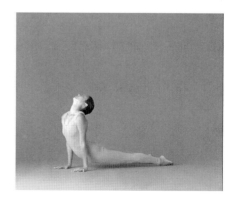

9. Exhale and let your legs pull you backward into Downward-Facing Dog.

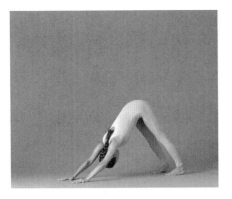

10. Breathe in Downward-Facing Dog, three to five breaths.

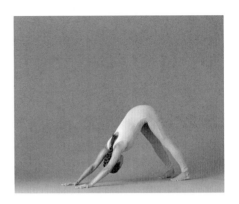

11. Exhale, and then at the bottom of your exhalation, reach your right foot forward into Lunge.

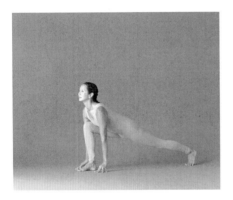

12. Inhale, extend and expand Lunge.

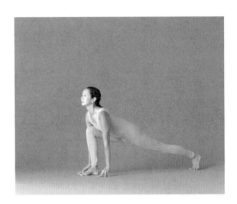

13. Exhale, and then at the bottom of your exhalation, step your left foot forward into Extended Standing Forward Bend.

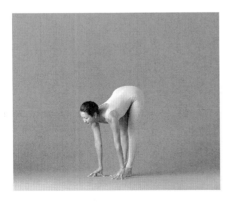

14. Inhale in Extended Standing Forward Bend.

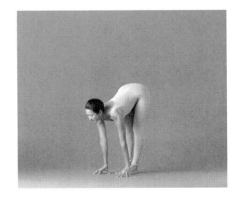

15. Exhale and release into Standing Forward Bend.

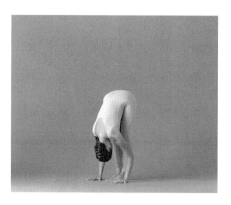

16. Inhale and rise up into Powerful Pose.

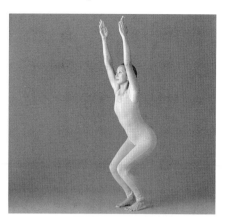

17. Exhale in Powerful Pose.

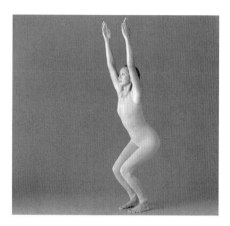

18. Inhale and rise up into Volcano Pose.

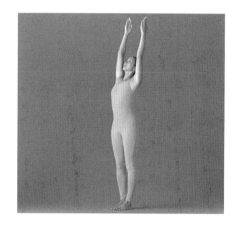

19. Exhale and release your arms into Mountain Pose.

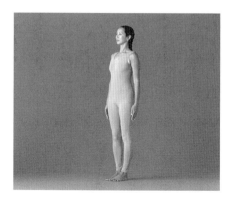

Second Salutation

Repeat the entire series on your left side. This means using your left foot instead of the right to reach back into Lunge and using your left foot to reach forward to return to Lunge.

Let this second Sun Salutation be a *graceful* practice. How can you explore grace in these poses? By gliding on your breath and feeling an organic coordination. By letting the vibrancy of your body ring completely. By sensing the organic undulations rising and echoing through your being.

Third Salutation

Repeat the entire series once again on the right side.

Let this third Sun Salutation be an *earthy* practice. How can you explore earthiness in these poses? By bringing your awareness to your contact with the ground. By feeling the pulsation of your feet and hands as they touch the earth. By letting the energy from the planet be drawn up through your feet and hands into the core of your heart.

Fourth Salutation

Repeat the entire series once again on the left side.

Let this fourth Sun Salutation be an *alignment* practice. How can you explore alignment in these poses? By letting your bones carry the weight of your body, so your muscles can be supple for freedom of movement and circulation. By using your muscles to move your body *through* your bones. By bearing your weight in the center of each limb and beginning to move with a relaxed sense of center.

Part 3: Extending the Salutation

You can intuitively extend the Sun Salutation to include more poses. Typically you insert these additional poses in the sequence after either the first or second lunge. Try this:

1. Repeat your Sun Salutation on the right side.

2. From the second Lunge, ground your back foot and move into Triangle Pose on the right side.

3. From Triangle Pose, return to Lunge.

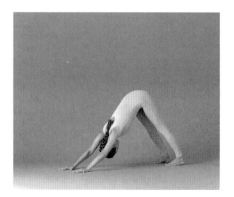

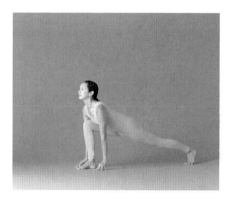

4. From Lunge, return to Downward-Facing Dog.

5. From Downward-Facing Dog, move your left foot forward into Lunge.

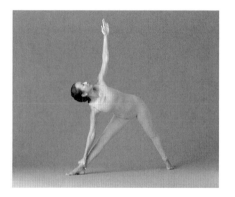

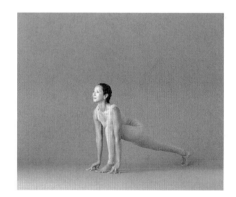

6. From Lunge, ground your back foot and move into Triangle Pose on the left side.

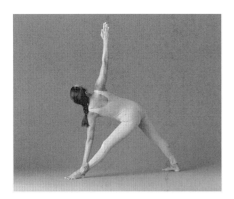

7. From Triangle Pose, move back to Lunge.

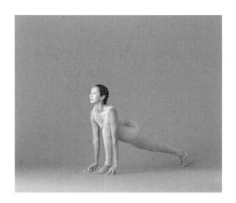

8. From Lunge, come back to Extended Standing Forward Bend.

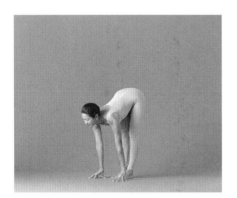

9. Complete the Sun Salutation as usual.

You can add Side Angle Pose, Warrior Pose 1, and Warrior Pose 2 to the sequence in the same manner.

Part 4: Relaxation Pose and Meditation

1. Relaxation Pose
5 to 10 minutes

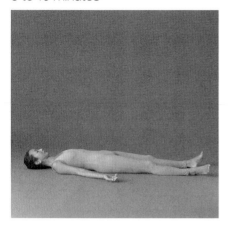

Instructions. As you situate yourself in Relaxation Pose, let go of all the gross movements of your body and begin to feel your *internal* stirrings: the pulse of your heart, the workings of your digestive tract, the waves of your breath, and the movement of relaxation in your muscular body.

One Thing. Feel like you are gazing into a tidal pool after a wave has receded. As your outer movements become still, allow yourself to observe the internal life in the flickering light (tiny fish and crabs swimming and darting about in chaotic abandon).

2. Sitting Meditation
5 minutes or intuition

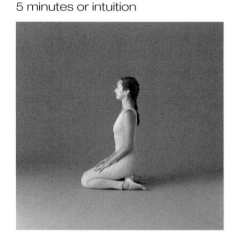

Sitting. Sit in Hero Pose, on a prop that is high enough for you to be stable and at ease. What does it mean to sit still? Isn't it movement that allows for stillness? Like flowing with the river instead of resisting it? Like allowing your body to move with the river of the present moment?

Your body should be fluidly rising and falling with your breath. Consciously move your posture—play with your posture—to become aware of your center. Move your arms. Re-place your hands. Shift the position of your head. Rock the placement of your pelvis. Undulate the alignment of your spine.

(If you wish to meditate longer than five minutes, come out of Hero Pose and assume your traditional seated position for meditation.)

Meditating. Watch the movement of your thoughts. Use your breath as a point of reference. When your mind wanders—when you observe it wandering—embrace it and bring it back to your breath.

Reconsidering the Practice

Our sedentary lifestyle not only debilitates our external bodies, but it walls in and crushes our inner movements. So enliven your muscular, skeletal body. Reignite the nature of your legs and the swing of your arms. And at the same time, let there be enough external quietness to allow:

the passions of your blood
the movements of your intestines
the sloshing of your fluids
the ruminations of your mind

Just play with movement—conscious movement, observed movement. Delight in the beauty of it. Immerse yourself in the sensation of it. (We are all somewhat inhibited in our body movements in this culture, but why not challenge yourself to break free of the shackles of conventionality?)

FIRST RIVER

In the beginning, it wasn't a river but a road, a road where there used to be a river, a river that led to the sea and then a curving road that led away, away from that place, and there were houses along the road, so many different sizes and colors of houses where the sycamore trees had been, sycamore trees that drank the fresh, clear water that was now a road along the riverbed, and this was where we lived, on that road, in a house that wasn't a sycamore tree, and smooth, round river stones, silvery white and silvery gray, were in the dry, sandy dirt, and I dug them up with broken branches and with my hands, and they were precious gems, and then what I remember was that a fire came and it burned the hills so bare that only a few sticks were left in the ground and the sticks crumbled when I touched them and made black marks on my hands, and then there was rain and rain and rain, and nothing left to hold down the dirt, and that was why the mud started, yellow-brown mud that people were afraid of, and it came out of the hills, the hills with only a few black sticks in them, and people were out in the rain at night, digging and digging the mud, all night long, and filling up bags and piling up bags and shouting, but it was too late, too late, and the rain kept coming and the yellow-brown mud that people were so afraid of kept coming, and in the morning I went to see and there it was: the river, a rushing, churning, yellow-brown river where there used to be a curving road, and I stood there so glad in white plastic rain boots.

— NINA ZOLOTOW

Sun Salutation Summary

1. Breathe in
Mountain Pose.

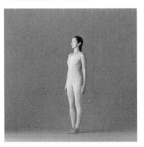

2. Inhale into
Volcano Pose.

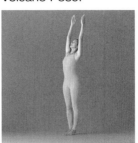

3. Exhale into Standing Forward Bend.

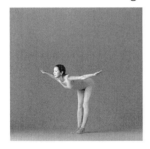
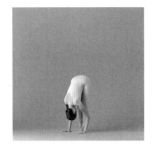

4. Inhale into Extended
Standing Forward
Bend.

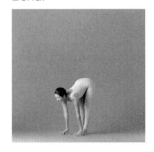

5. Exhale into Lunge.

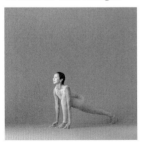

6. Inhale and expand
Lunge.

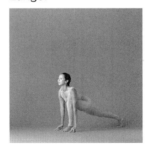

7. Exhale into Plank Pose or Push-up Pose.

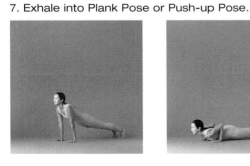

8. Inhale into Upward-
Facing Dog.

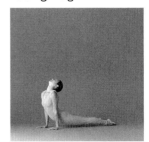

9. Exhale into
Downward-Facing Dog.

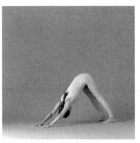

10. Breathe in
Downward-Facing Dog.

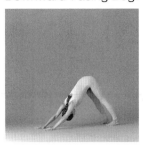

11. Exhale into Lunge.

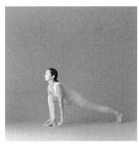

12. Inhale and expand
Lunge.

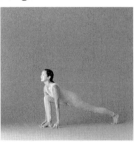

13. Exhale into
Extended Standing
Forward Bend.

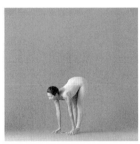

14. Inhale in Extended
Standing Forward
Bend.

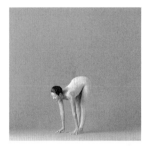

15. Exhale into Standing
Forward Bend.

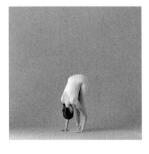

16. Inhale into Powerful
Pose.

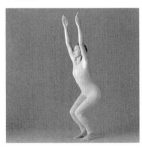

17. Exhale in Powerful
Pose.

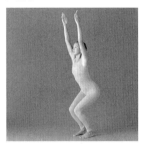

18. Inhale into Volcano
Pose.

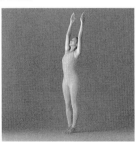

19. Exhale into
Mountain Pose.

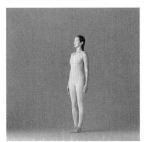

True Confessions

NINA   You're falling asleep.

ROD   No, I'm contemplating. I would just like to go around and ask people who they think God is. And what spirituality is, for that matter.

NINA   That's an issue for me because I come from a background that actively rejects anything of that kind. I always say that I am a third-generation atheist because the grandparent I was closest to was my maternal grandmother, who grew up in an Orthodox Jewish family in a small village in Lithuania, and she rejected all of that. It goes that far back in my family. So it's very difficult for me to be a person who can even admit—and I'm getting there very slowly—that I'm engaging in a spiritual practice, because of the—

ROD   Who says this is a spiritual practice?

NINA   I do. Now.

ROD   Oh my God, you've gotten further than I have.

NINA   Right.

ROD   I have no idea what people talk about when they use the word *spiritual*.

NINA   Well, I can talk about what I mean. You know, we've made some progress in our discussions, and I've thought a lot and I've read a lot, and I've even read our discussions over and over while I was working on them, and I have come to the conclusion that yoga does affect my experience of life. You remember, we went through this long discussion where I ended up by saying that yoga made me feel happier about being alive, that it made me feel more connected to life. This was after you pushed on me really hard, after you kept on asking me, "And what does *feeling good* mean?" Do you remember that?

ROD   Yes, I remember it clearly.

NINA   I've been working on it ever since then. My friend Melitta and I talk about these things all the time—why we do yoga and what it does or doesn't do for us. We go out for tea after class, and she's even cried a couple of times. There we are, sitting in Gaylord's Cafe, and she's crying and talking about how yoga has helped her deal with the deeper emotional effects of having diabetes. You know, how it has helped her cope with living with an incurable illness.

ROD   So what do you think spirituality is, by the way?

NINA   Well, what I'm saying is simply that for me doing yoga has something to do with my well-being as a person.

ROD   This is interesting. If I ask myself that question—what is spirituality?—I feel like I can't make the distinction at all. I feel like, oh my God, it's everything.

NINA   That's fair enough.

ROD   Maybe the word *spirituality* deals with a component of our being that's not as tangible as a physical part of our body but is nonetheless as real. But it's hard to say where physicality ends and spirituality begins. As I practice yoga and delve more deeply into my physical body, I tend to get confused about what the physical body is. What are atoms of the physical body? And what are atoms of spirituality?

NINA   Well, that's fine. I don't disagree with that. But for me, I had a lot of resistance to using that word.

ROD   Right, right. I couldn't agree with you more. I have a hard time using that word myself. *Spirituality.* I fall into it every so often, but it's not something that feels easy slipping off my tongue.

NINA   True confessions . . .

ROD   I think it's the way it's used—like a sleight of hand type of thing. If I really listen to people when they use that word, it's like a big flag that denotes patriotism or something. It's like, oh, they're spiritual because they believe in something, and everyone else who doesn't believe in that something is somehow *not* spiritual. It's like, oh wow, that really makes me feel holistic. Let's divide things even more into spiritual and nonspiritual. So tell me, is the mind spiritual and the body not spiritual? Are human beings the only things with spirit? How about animals and plants and rocks and planets and stars? Where's the dividing line? Who's making the rules?

NINA   The other day a friend of mine said, "You don't do yoga for spiritual reasons, right?" And I said, "Well, actually I do."

ROD   [laughs] Oh my God, I wish I would have been there.

NINA   He seemed very disappointed in me. He said, "*What?*"

ROD   Nina, you have fallen to the monster! You fell to the monster. What are we going to do?

NINA   I know, I know. I'm falling into yoga—

ROD   This is a funny conversation. I sort of like it. You're falling to the monster.

NINA   [laughs] Okay, now you can talk about how good it is to not be stuck in one place.

ROD   What do you mean, "not be stuck in one place"?

NINA   Oh, stuck in one belief or one point of view.

ROD   Right. You're movable, Nina. You're changing—right before my very eyes. But how does it *feel* to shift your beliefs? Is it scary? Is it exciting? Does it feel like there's any sense of loss?

NINA   It does make me feel a bit queasy sometimes, because it's like I'm turning into a kind of person I never expected to be. However, it's also a big relief. Because it can be pretty boring to go through your whole life being what you expect to be.

ROD   Yeah, to me, at first moving feels unfamiliar, but it also feels more alive. So maybe the trick is to know that you're always moving and to keep on observing that movement. Maybe we can even feel secure with not having strong beliefs, and that it's not a sign of weakness that we shift our belief system. And we might even conclude that if we *stop* moving, we're living in an illusion that we've created out of a need for security, in fear of the unknown. The Buddhists have an idea of impermanence. Maybe our identities and our belief systems are just as impermanent as anything else. So instead of finding a new orientation to hold on to and cement into place, maybe we can bring all of our faculties into being present with the movement.

So any more true confessions, Nina? Did I win any more arguments?

NINA   Okay, I might as well come clean completely. Just a few days ago, I wrote to a friend something like this: "My yoga teacher has always been asking me whether yoga makes me feel more emotionally balanced, and until lately I always said no. Lately I decided that I do feel emotionally balanced, and that this was partly because I'd redefined the term. So I can still be on anti-depressants, and get insomnia attacks, and feel horribly homesick when I travel, and all that, but who's to say that's not emotionally balanced? I've just decided that it's all fine."

ROD   God, Nina, how amazing to hear you stop defining yourself and caging yourself with an idea of being emotionally balanced! Where did that initial idea come from anyway? It really is wonderful to hear that you can accept who you are at this time and see that as a type of balance, as a form of balance. When I go into the forest, I see trees of all different shapes and forms, like beautiful, artistic bonsai trees. They all have a natural, intrinsic balance. And furthermore, in context with all the other trees in their surroundings, they couldn't be more perfect in their shape.

NINA   But don't you think what I said might be rather shocking to people? Don't you think it's a pretty radical statement?

ROD   By all means. And it's going to be shocking to people partly because they might think that this leads to being apathetic. That accepting yourself might not lead to desired change. But in fact, my experience is that acceptance of yourself is the *foundation* for understanding and being immersed in change.

But anyway, I can't believe you're admitting this! All your old friends might dump you, thinking you've turned into a New Age mental wimp.

NINA   Oh, no, then I'll have to be friends with all you yoga people!

ROD   Well, just think about my predicament! I don't have anyone to argue with anymore. You keep agreeing with me.

But honestly, I feel like I'm becoming less and less stable myself. I really don't see the fascination at all with holding on. This letting go has given me more enjoyment in the last year. I feel like I have more and more freedom to show up and be who I am at a given moment. I feel it's easier for me to suspend my own ideas and relax with what other people are saying to me. It's really quite intriguing to let another person's feelings and thoughts and physical sensations be received as your own. I actually believe this is the beginning of understanding and compassion.

Being Present

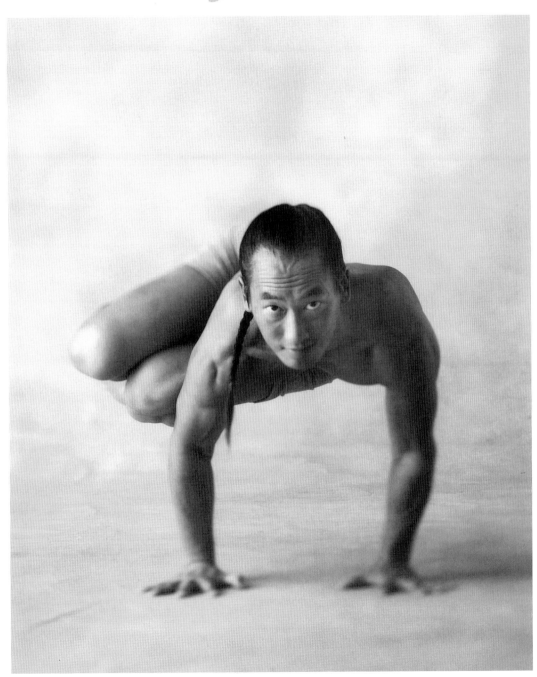

THE RED WHEELBARROW

So much depends
upon

a red wheel
barrow

glazed with rain
water

beside the white
chickens.

— WILLIAM CARLOS WILLIAMS

Take Me with You

NINA   The last time my whole family was together, my husband was teasing my brother about how he used to hate it when we were kids and I sat alone on the couch reading. Because I would get so completely absorbed in my book that I would ignore everything that was going on around me, and if anyone in my family started talking to me, I didn't even hear them. It wasn't that I was intentionally ignoring them, but I was just so completely lost in my own world. And it used to drive my brother absolutely crazy. He would stand there dropping marbles on top of me or doing anything he could think of to get my attention. And the extraordinary thing is that he's *still* upset about it. When my husband started teasing him last week, my brother—who's forty-five now—started getting angry about it all over again, and I finally asked him, "I don't understand—why are you still so mad at me about that?"

And he said, "Don't you see? You had this way of getting completely away, of escaping from the bad things that were going on in our everyday life, and *you didn't take me with you.*"

It was quite moving, actually. He sounded sad and even a little bitter. *"You didn't take me with you."* But I thought, "How could I? How could I take you with me?"

ROD   Well, that's why people have gurus. They want someone to take them with them. You know, save my soul, take me to a place where I don't have to feel this difficulty. And it may happen for a while, but then you realize you're right back in it. It cycles back around, and you need another fix of some kind. It's like, "This is an endless cycle and I can't get off." Everybody wants to get off. That's in a lot of your stories: stop the world, I want to get off!

And at some point in that cycle, there's an excruciating scream because there's an excruciating, infinite pain at the very seat of your soul. It's so amazingly painful that all you can be is in complete, sheer arrest. And then for whatever reason it dissipates. It's like that poem you gave me by Jane Kenyon about anger:

> So it is when we retreat in anger:
> we think we burn alone
> and there is no balm.
> Then water enters, though it makes
> no sound.

Where did that come from? Is it you? Is it something you decided? Is it someone else? Is it yoga? Is it medicine? Is it pain relievers? Is it God? Is it your fairy godmother? Is it your guardian angel? Is it the spirit of your grandmother? Is it some Native American chief? Is it some Chinese sage? Is it some Jewish mystic? Is it some South American shaman? Is it some African medicine man? Is it the words of Aristotle or Socrates? What the hell is it? What's going to get you out of this?

Observing Your Breath

IN AND OUT

The dog searches until he finds me
upstairs, lies down with a clatter
of elbows, puts his head on my foot.

Sometimes the sound of his breathing
saves my life—in and out, in
and out; a pause, a long sigh. . . .

— JANE KENYON

What a relief to be able to spend part of your day *not doing*. To simply lie back and take in your breath. And observe one of the most fundamental aspects of your aliveness. It's like stargazing. Your mind wanders a bit—then you see the stars—then your mind wanders again—then you see another part of the night sky. Watching your breath can be that mesmerizing, and before you know it you've become part of something larger than the confines of your habitual consciousness.

The time you spend observing your breath will not only restore you physically but will add depth and dimension to your life. Because by its very nature your breath brings you into the present moment. For it is always what is happening to you now. And its ever-changing quality brings you to a visceral understanding of impermanence. That knowledge can help you let go of your obsessions with the past and your longings and worries about the future so you can experience fully what is happening to you today, in this place, in this hour, in this minute, with this breath.

It's not so easy to observe your breath, but it can be like looking at a great painting. Every day you can see something new in it—colors, brush strokes, emotions. Partly it's a matter of understanding the relationship between breath and relaxation. Have you ever noticed how as someone is just about to fall asleep, his breath shifts, taking on a more prominent quality? In a breath observation practice, you are trying to get into that same state of deep relaxation while still remaining conscious. It's like learning how to see all those odd fish in the deepest, darkest part of the sea—you need to be able to drop that far down into your own ocean. When it's that quiet, you can begin to see your breath.

Breath Observation Exercises

Remember playing with your breath when you were a kid? Remember blowing bubbles when you were learning to swim? Remember how you and your friends would plunge underwater to see who could hold their breath the longest? Remember underwater tea parties? Remember holding your breath as your parents drove through a tunnel, so you could get your wish?

This section provides seven breath observation exercises for you to try. These games provide backgrounds against which you can observe the organic rising of your breath the way you can see the movements of clouds against the sky. Bring a sense of curiosity to these breath games.

Practicing

We suggest that for one week you do one breath exercise per day, starting with the first exercise on the first day and finishing with the seventh exercise on the seventh day. Then repeat the entire cycle three times over three more weeks.

We recommend a structured program because if you try to be intuitive from the start, you will probably fall *into* your habit instead of *out of* your habit, because your habit will feel like intuition. But by putting yourself into a program of breath awareness that is not your own, you get a chance to play someone else's game, which might give you a closer look at who you are. And from there—a place of questioning—you can start to be more intuitive about what practices you might want to do every day. (Actually, if you get this far—having practiced a full month of breath observation—we recommend that you turn to a yoga teacher in your area for further instruction.)

If you can't manage to practice every day, don't worry. Just practice as often as you can, but realize that unless you approach this practice with a certain level of consistency, the subtleties of your breath will not be revealed.

You don't need to be in a monastery to do these exercises. Simply find a quiet area where you feel comfortable, and set aside fifteen to thirty minutes a day when there is nothing distracting you. Be willing to let nothing interrupt you—simply decide that nothing will take precedence over your breath practice. It's also best to do the exercises when you are already quiet and calm, and at least two hours after eating. Most practitioners find that first thing in the morning, before breakfast, is the best time (sorry, but yes, you do have to get out of bed). If you end up doing it in the middle of your daily activities, start with a restorative pose first, such as Relaxation Pose, Legs Up the Wall Pose, or Reclined Cobbler's Pose with a bolster.

Try to figure out how you are going to fit this into your life. Most people who make it work end up being pragmatic—doing it at the same time every day. Give it a chance. Do it on faith for six months, without questioning. Because ultimately it will make a profound difference in your life.

Precautions

If any of these exercises cause any physical, emotional, or mental irritations or difficulties while you are practicing (for example, watering eyes, ringing in the ears, twitches in the nervous system, irritability, or shakiness), return to basic Relaxation Pose in any of its variations.

Never force or hold your breath. Trying to alter your breath before you can observe it deeply is like trying to defuse a bomb before you understand what all the wires do. Your first task is simply to learn about the wiring of your body that's currently in place. What are your habitual patterns? For example, ask yourself what muscles you contract when you breathe, where your breath moves easily, or which parts of your body you associate with and which parts you are not even conscious of.

Relaxing

You will do all these breath observation exercises while in various forms of Relaxation Pose. After making your initial adjustments in the pose to create as much symmetry and ease as possible, make a final decision not to make any more adjustments. From then on, if you notice a restriction, an irritation, or an obstacle, don't move. Just focus on the restriction and ask yourself: can I simply observe the gripping and the releasing?

We're used to creating new tensions to compensate for tensions that we let go of; conscious relaxation may allow the tension to leave the whole body-mind rather than just shifting it around from one place to another. But as we're letting go of tension, we come to unfamiliar places, and feelings of uneasiness are not unusual as we move toward emptiness.

What is the state of mind between sleep and wakefulness, where you are still conscious, maybe even superconscious, of the thoughts and feelings in yourself and the room but where you are detached from the need to interact and respond? This is the foundation state for your breath observation, which is the essence of a breath practice.

Observing

Effort and tension often show up as tightness in the skin of your face or your sense organs and are indications that there is not enough relaxation and surrender. So in exercises where you are observing your breath, put equal importance on observing the waves of tension and effort in your face.

Absorbing Your Breath

What's the feeling when you have intimacy with someone? You'll have that same feeling when you allow your breath to be fully absorbed. To lose yourself in the smell of your lover's neck— that's what your breath practice can be. A practice where you are being that intimate with yourself. . . .

Breath Game 1:
Observation of Your Breath
in Your Body

Timing. 20 minutes.

Relaxation Pose. For this exercise, lie in Classic Relaxation Pose, as described on page 316. Keep a folded blanket nearby (fold the blanket into quarters, and then fold it one more time into a long rectangle).

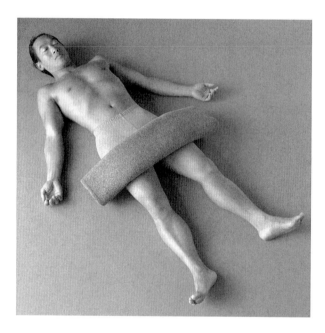

Step 1 (2 to 3 minutes). Lying in Relaxation Pose, place the blanket on your thighs. Feel your thighs relax as the weight of the blanket helps focus your attention on them. This sustained attention in and of itself will allow you to let go more. As you truly relax your legs, you begin to let go of the fight-or-flight mechanism in your body, and your legs will return to being streams of light from your belly.

Step 2 (2 to 3 minutes). Place the blanket on your belly. Notice the great fluctuations there—this is

the beginning of the waves that ripple from your center to the ends of your extremities. When you are quiet, your breath sets up a wave in your body, which ripples through your skin, your bones, and your muscles. A resonance. A vibration. Like throwing a stone in a pond.

Step 3 (2 to 3 minutes). Place the blanket on your lower ribs. Notice the nature of the direction of movement of your lower ribs underneath the blanket. Picture the breath of a sleeping baby—the suppleness of its chest. Ask yourself: What am I scared of? Why am I gripping the natural movements of my lower ribs? Your lower ribs should feel as though they are spreading like the wings of a bird drying the wetness of the morning from its feathers. Allow them to spread to your sides as your mind drops downward to your heart.

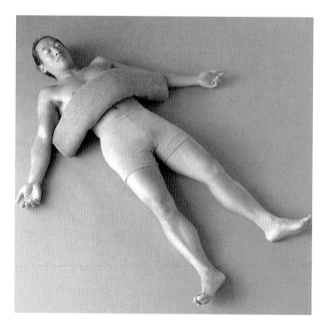

Step 4 (2 to 3 minutes). Place the blanket on your upper ribs. The skin on your upper chest is like a gossamer veil over your soul. It softens the light that touches your heart. As you observe your breath, become aware of the tender movements of your upper chest, without any effort in your throat or face. Be completely absorbed in this most ethereal of all movements.

Step 5 (2 to 3 minutes). Place the blanket over your eyes and forehead. Feel a willingness to let go into not knowing, into sadness, into the sigh, into the fragility, into the longing. Observe the skin of your forehead drop toward your eyes, your eyebrows releasing wide toward your temples, and the skin of your temples dropping toward the back of your skull. And feel your eyes deepening in their sockets, like lustrous pearls falling into soft sand as the warm ocean waters of your breath envelop them.

Let the air swirl around in your nose, swirl around in your body, and swirl around in your mind. Like a drop of color falling into clear water. As you begin to stir it, watch the thick, viscous color slowly dissolve until it permeates every particle of clear water.

Relaxing Afterward (5 minutes). As you lie in Relaxation Pose, let go of focusing on specific areas and feel your entire body rising and falling.

Breath Game 2:
The Direction of Your Breath

Timing. 20 minutes.

Relaxation Pose. For this exercise, lie in Relaxation Pose on a bolster, with a folded blanket under your head, as shown. If your lower back hurts, you can place a blanket roll under your legs.

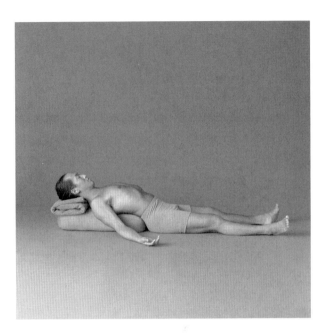

Observing (5 minutes). How much can you relax your legs and arms and feel the relationship between that relaxation and the course and depth of your breath? Can you decipher the direction of the flow of your breath? Following a breath is like following a thread in a weaving. So follow the threads of your breath—see how they are moving in your body. If you have places that don't move easily with your breath, those areas might be laden with emotion, trauma, or difficulty. As you make your way into them, your breath doesn't always elicit a memory, but it can elicit a release.

Inhaling (5 minutes). In general, observe how your inhalation enters through your nose and flows to the back of your skull and down the front of your spine into the depths of your groins. It is not through your effort or determination but through the relaxation of your legs that your inhalation is drawn into your body. As your legs and arms get heavier and heavier, more space is created in your torso, producing a deeper vacuum in your body. Relaxation can become the source of the deepening of your inhalation.

When a waterfall falls from the top of a cliff to the depths of a crater, the water draws air down with it. And as the water and air cascade down the cliff, the water begins to fill up the crater. *This is your inhalation.*

So can you feel that the pool of water is your belly and that the waterfall is the moist air moving through your nose? Observe it as it moves down through your lungs and abdomen to the pit of your belly and into the depth of your groins. Feel it slowly rising through your groins, wavering your abdominal skin and broadening into your lower ribs to the expanse of your middle and upper chest.

Exhaling (5 minutes). In general, observe how your exhalation moves in the direction of your upper sternum from the source of your groins. The relaxation follows your exhalation, moving from your legs to the crown of your head. As your entire being relaxes more, your exhalation will drop even further toward emptiness.

When the water in the mountain lake evaporates into the sky, it moves upward, slowly emptying the crater that contains it. As you exhale, your chest stays expansive as the volume of air slowly decreases—the volume of air is moving up but emptying down. *This is your exhalation.*

As you exhale, can you feel that the breath keeps streaming from the front of your tailbone through your back lower ribs and out the top of your sternum? Notice how the direction of the breath helps maintain the expansiveness of the chest until the very end of your exhalation. Sense how the exhalation releases you into union.

Relaxing Afterward (5 minutes). As you lie in Relaxation Pose, observe how both your inhalation and your exhalation allow you to release your tensions into the earth.

Breath Game 3:
Directing Your Inhalation

Timing. 20 minutes.

Relaxation Pose. For this exercise, lie in Relaxation Pose with your calves on a chair, as shown.

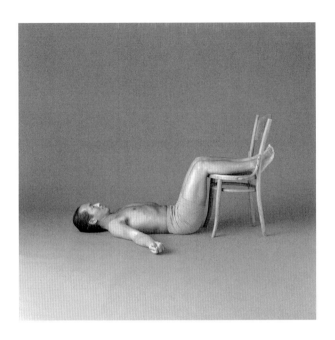

Directing Your Breath. By "directing" your breath, we mean observe what is already occurring and enhance it with a light intention. Do you think that you only breathe into your lungs? *When you take in a breath, your whole body is getting oxygen through all the capillaries—inhaling into all the living tissues of your body and your mind.*

Step 1 (5 minutes). Place your hands on your belly. Observe the watery rising and falling of this area, and notice how the absorption of your inhalation increases as you completely drop everything except your observation. Feel the depth of the cavity of your pelvis, and explore this cavern with the sound and feel of your breath.

Step 2 (5 minutes). Feel your back lower ribs on the ground. Direct your breath into this area with your awareness but not with muscular force or hard intention. Sense how your lower ribs absorb your breath and broaden along the ground like syrup being poured on a buttermilk pancake. Observe the spaces between your ribs and the expansion of those spaces as you inhale.

Step 3 (5 minutes). Notice how the back of your head is resting on the ground. Feel your eyes soften, the root of your tongue soften, the bridge of your nose widen, the skin of your face become more receptive, and your ears deepen. On your inhalation, relax all of your sense organs deeper into your skull as you direct your inhalation into the cavity at the back of your skull. Keep following a conscious dream of someone caressing the back of your head.

Relaxing Afterward (5 minutes). As you lie in Relaxation Pose, continue to notice and observe any resistance to the absorption of your breath on your inhalations.

Breath Game 4:
Completing Your Exhalations

Timing. 20 minutes.

Relaxation Pose. For this exercise, lie in Classic Relaxation Pose with no props.

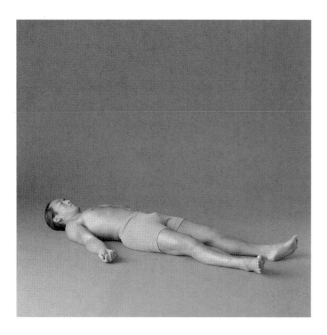

Observing Your Exhalations (10 minutes). Start by observing the quality of your exhalations. Notice how your body and mind naturally relax their tension and dissipate their holding as you exhale. As your exhalation comes to its finish, do you notice the pause, a moment of complete stillness, right before you inhale? How does your body react to this silence? Are you anxious to inhale?

Feeling. Feel the slow tapering of your breath into the void. Linger in the essence of emptiness as you would with the fragrance of a flower. *The last trails of the fingers of light receding into night.*

Elongating the Pauses (5 minutes). Now that you've explored the natural pauses at the base of your exhalations, begin to intuitively elongate those pauses so they last from one to three seconds. These moments of deep surrender at the bottom of your exhalations will bring you to profound rest.

Relaxing Afterward (5 minutes). As you lie in Relaxation Pose, notice your unmanipulated, habitual exhalations. How do they compare with your previous elongated exhalations? Which seem more relaxing?

Breath Game 5:
Regulating Your Inhalation and Exhalation

Timing. 20 minutes.

Relaxation Pose. For this exercise, lie in Relaxation Pose on a bolster with a folded blanket under your head, as shown. Place a folded blanket on your thighs—let its weight help bring your awareness to this area of your body.

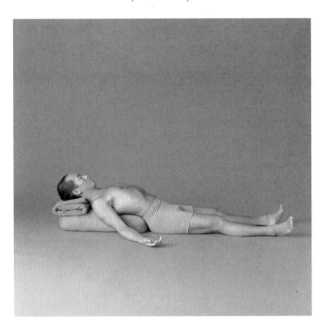

Metering Your Breath (5 minutes). As you observe your inhalations and exhalations, begin to meter their length by counting them—not to change them but just to observe them. Which is longer? Which is smoother? With which do you feel more at ease?

Meter your breath not to harness it like a horse but to *unbridle* it. Simply observe its raw beauty and vibrancy. Let it put you in a state of awe and return your mind to a state of not knowing and wonderment.

Regulating Your Breath (10 minutes). Now try to make your inhalation and exhalation of equal length by shortening the one that is longer. There is a natural underlying rhythm that modulates continuously. Let your breath fall into that natural rhythm at the same time that you regulate it, so that equalizing your inhalation and exhalation draws you deeper into equanimity.

When to Stop. If regulating your breath causes any physical or mental irritation, allow yourself to return to mere observation of your breath. Let your breath lead you into deepening your relaxation.

Relaxing Afterward (5 minutes). As you lie in Relaxation Pose, return to simple observation of your breath. It might be difficult at this point to observe without manipulating, but continue to practice letting go of the tendency to control.

Breath Game 6:
Opening the Architecture of Your Chest

Timing. 20 minutes.

Relaxation Pose. For this exercise, lie in Classic Relaxation Pose, as shown. Keep a blanket that is folded into quarters and rolled into a tight roll nearby. (If your lower back is irritated during this exercise, try alternating between straight, dropped open legs, and bent legs.

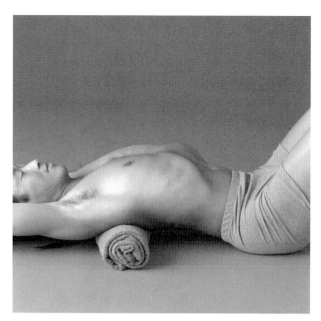

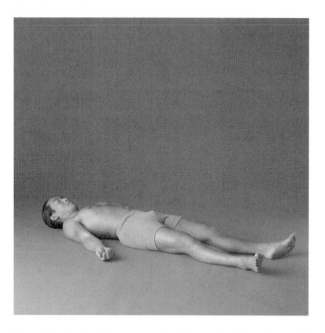

Step 1 (2 to 3 minutes). Place the blanket roll under your upper back, so the middles of your shoulder blades are on the apex of the roll. Make sure the roll is not too big so that as it supports your back it doesn't irritate your neck (if it does, place a pillow under your head). Now breathe into your upper back muscles so they widen from your spine. As you breathe into this area, feel not only how your upper back opens but also how the support of your back opens your upper front chest so it feels like a spinnaker sail. Let the base of your neck be unleashed from this broadness.

Step 2 (2 to 3 minutes). Place the blanket roll under your back lower ribs. Feel how your back lower ribs widen along the blanket with your in-halation. This lift to your back lower ribs also supports your front lower ribs. But as you breathe, focus on the broadening out of your side lower ribs, not on the lifting up of your front lower ribs. Allow any bindings to be unlaced.

Step 3 (2 to 3 minutes). Make the blanket roll slightly thinner (by unrolling part of it) and place it under your lower back. Ensure that it is small enough to provide support for your lower back without irritation. As you breathe into this area, let any knots and pain in your lower back dissipate into the natural pliability of your lower spine. Undo all your habitual bracing, realizing that suppleness is stronger than rigidity.

Step 4 (2 to 3 minutes). Roll the blanket back to full size and place it under your sacrum. As you breathe into this area, feel how soothing and yet exhilarating it is to be supported and lifted under your sacrum. This is your center—your sacred bone. Feel your breath spread into the broadness of your sacrum. The fragrance of the outside world enters your body slowly, beginning to spread like watercolor on fine paper, inking every absorbent fiber of your body.

Step 5 (2 to 3 minutes). Place the blanket roll under your legs. Now come back into full rest, feeling your entire back torso touching the earth, the totality of your back body receiving your breath while at the same time supporting the expanse of your chest. Be sensitive to your entire back body in its chaotic, undulating movements, like a magic carpet riding on the currents of the air.

Relaxing Afterward (5 minutes). As you lie in Relaxation Pose, observe your torso. As you notice your habitual posture begin to creep back in and encase your vulnerability to create the illusion of security, see if you can break those habits and drop into new, subtle states of relaxation.

Breath Game 7:
Allowing Deeper Breaths

Timing. 20 minutes.

Relaxation Pose. For this exercise, lie in Relaxation Pose over a bolster, with a folded blanket or pillow under your head, as shown.

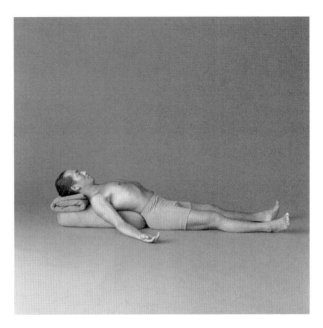

Relaxing. When you take off your shoes and walk around in summer flip-flops, your feet are happy to be unlaced from the prison of your winter shoes. As you lie on the bolster, feel how your body naturally wants to open to a deeper breath. Allow your legs to fall a little farther from the height of your chest, creating a larger vacuum within your body, which invites a more absorbed and complete breath.

Absorbing Your Breath (5 minutes). The intention here is to take not a bigger breath but a more absorbed breath that seems to be drawn into every cell of your body. It is as though you were letting go of the armor around your vulnerability, your body-mind completely acknowledging its thirst for the divine nectar of your breath. Surrender to its taste, to its fragrance. Begin to take slow, smooth breaths, breathing through your nose as if you were taking long sips of air.

Taking a Complete Breath (10 minutes). As you inhale into the direction of your groins, take long, slow, smooth inhalations that move from your side lower ribs up to your middle ribs and then to your upper ribs. During the inhalation, make sure your facial muscles and your sense organs relax deeply. If there is any noticeable tension, make your inhalations shorter, because smoothness is more important than length. In fact, it is not advisable to go to your limits — stay well within your boundaries. *The inhalation is the movement from the ether to the earth, from the universal consciousness into the individual consciousness.*

As you exhale in the direction of your sternum, allow your belly to recede first, eliciting a smooth release of your chest cavity throughout the length of your exhalation. During your exhalation, feel your entire being dropping to the earth, and the boundaries of your mind expanding. Spend the time at the bottom of your exhalation to feel it tapering more and more toward emptiness. *The exhalation is the movement from the earth toward the ether, from individual consciousness to universal consciousness.*

Relaxing Afterward (5 minutes). As you lie in Relaxation Pose, scan your body in observation, from the soles of your feet to the crown of your head.

Fall in love with your breath.

Rewiring the Body

ROD So, Nina, do you think your relationships have improved through your practice of yoga? Go out on a limb here with me. I mean do you think yoga has improved your main relationships, like your marriage, your relationship with your children, your relationship with your main friends?

NINA I *am* trying to use some of the ideas to be more patient and get less swept away by my emotions with my family—you know, just to be there with them. I am consciously working with it. But no miracles have occurred.

ROD To me what you're saying about not getting swept away with your emotions and being able to stay with the present moment no matter what's happening is something I relate directly to yoga. Certain relationships of mine—profound relationships, like my relationship with my father— changed drastically, I think, through the practice. I believe we're not so different from Pavlov's dog—you know, a bell rings and the dog salivates. And I think we all have a lot of habits like that in our body. The phone rings and your nervous system comes to attention—oh, I have to answer that. Now we've retrained ourselves with the answering machines—now it's, oh, I can wait and listen. But I remember the times my body used to jump. I would be in Relaxation Pose and I would feel the knee-jerk response that I would have to a simple thing like a phone ringing. And then after a lot of yoga practice, I would be hearing the sound of the phone ringing without actually having a reaction to it. I could say, oh, that's the phone ringing. Should I answer it? My body wasn't actually reacting to it—there was a choice at that point. And so something as simple as that shows me that the practice of yoga does have an amazing way of beginning to take your reactive body and bring you to this place where sounds are just sounds, and sight is just sight. And this detachment is the ability to see things as they are. And I think if you begin to see things more as they are and not as you want them to be or as you imagine them to be, you actually have the freedom to be in the present moment, and that is empowering.

To be completely present in the moment with all your faculties—with your emotions, with your mind, with your body, with your breath—means, in some sense, you're fully living your life because your life is happening now, the manifested life. In some sense I'm a pragmatist. Sure, I may believe in reincarnation, but the belief doesn't matter to me. What I know is that I'm alive now, and I feel more able to be alive in the moment because of the yoga practice.

NINA   What I do see sometimes is a new ability to get over things faster, like when you're a child and get over a fight with another little kid right away instead of hanging on to it all day. For example, when I have a fight with my husband, what I do is just try to let go of it and say I'm sorry. I just try to stop acting angry. So then, of course, he can let go, too. So I've been consciously putting that into practice. I don't think I've been that successful at stopping the knee-jerk reactions. There are certain things that set me off, like when he criticizes the way I do housework or he gets mad at me because he can't find something. That totally sets me off. You know, it's like you talking about your dad—

ROD   Yes—every time I used to get together with my dad there were certain things that sounded like a goddamned tape recorder. We'd get right into a specific kind of talk, and then it would be over in a couple of minutes— we'd be storming out of the room. After a while, I realized maybe my dad had a bad day or maybe it wasn't about me. His anger was not about me. His difficulty was not about me. His difficulty was with himself. So why should I get angry at that and make it even worse? Yoga basically changed my gut reaction to my father. My stomach didn't turn over. My heartbeat didn't get faster. My breath didn't clench up. All because I realized that I could relax—I could do Relaxation Pose while my dad was talking to me— so what's the big deal? If the phone can ring and I don't jump anymore, then my dad can talk to me and I can just sit and listen.

It was quite amazing to me that I changed my relationship with my father. Actually, I felt like I changed my relationship with myself. And since I didn't have a reaction, the entire chemical reaction was different. I mean basically it's like this in philosophy, if A plus B equals C, then if B changes, A plus B no longer equals C.

NINA   Right—it's like I can end a fight because I'm refusing to fight anymore, so he can't fight with me.

ROD   So the whole equation changes when one of the elements changes. So it's like fire and gunpowder make an explosion, but if you change the gunpowder to water, it's going to have a different outcome. So many years I thought, I need to change my dad. I need to make him understand me. And I finally realized that all I had to do was understand myself. Once I was fine with myself, then I was unshakable. The interesting thing is, as soon as I felt that way myself, he respected me as an adult.

NINA   You know, as you're talking I'm reminded of the theory of how therapy is supposed to work, by bringing your awareness to these things so you can stop being so caught up in them. But I'm not sure therapy actually works.

ROD   To me, it's not just awareness, and I think that's where regular therapy may fall short. And what I mean by that is, unless people are actually making an alchemical change in their bodies, literally beginning to deconstruct the neurological patterns that exist in the body, then I don't think just the awareness of something necessarily defuses it.
         In yoga the body is seen as a collection of the past, and in Western thought the body has what is called *kinetic memory*. For instance, let's say you go the same way to work every day and you take the same freeway exit. And let's say it's Saturday and you're not working.

NINA   Yeah, right. We've all done that.

ROD   But you end up—

NINA   You're on autopilot.

ROD   Yes, you end up taking the same exit because it's almost like a kinetic memory of the body. How do you remember how to ride a bicycle? Are you remembering how to ride it? No—it's a neurological memory, and your relationship with your parents or any past relationship also has a neurological memory. It's got a body memory to it. I think your body tends to say, oh, this is the way I am around this person. So what happens is that when a relationship gets stuck in a rut, the body keeps on having the same experience over and over again. Just like, oh, the bell rings, the dog is going to get food. So if enough times your husband makes some comment about the house not being clean and it causes this reaction in you, it actually builds the reaction deeper in your body. Yoga, to me, literally gets into the cellular body. It frees you of those connections, so you're not wired the same way anymore. It's literally rewiring the body.

NINA That would be nice.

ROD It happens. It's already happening to you. You're just too scared to admit it.

NINA Why do you think I'm scared of it?

ROD First of all, you're married to a scientist. And you have an analytical mind. I have an extremely analytical mind and I can always—with my analytical mind—deconstruct any argument for anything.

NINA For anything.

ROD You can basically say bullshit to anything. It's easy after a while. I can do it. I've done it all my life. I did it in my twenties until I was sick of myself. But I think the question is: why does the mind want to stay skeptical? What is it protecting itself from by remaining skeptical? For instance, when I first started yoga, I really had a hard time with bhakti yoga. Bhakti yoga is devotional, and I really couldn't understand why anyone would serve someone else as if they were a great channel to God. I thought that was really dangerous, but I have to say I'm more open to it now. I can see why people do it now, and I can see a usefulness in it, and I even admire it to a certain extent, that someone can surrender themselves to another person so much that they just allow themselves not to have doubt.

NINA Well, that's fair. I agree that there's an element of fear in my skepticism.

ROD And I think that's interesting to look at, that's all. I mean whether it's good, bad, or indifferent. But let's go back to another point that I heard you say that I think is interesting because I think yoga has really changed this for me. You said that you think that recently you've been able to—as you and your husband have gotten into arguments—let go of your point of view, maybe, and it doesn't matter who's right. To me, that's another thing that comes from yoga—this whole thing of defending your point of view and not being able to let go of your point of view begins to shift in yoga. I think that yoga actually begins to open your body and mind to realize, oh, there's a lot of point of views all the time and that maybe you can actually drop your point of view if, for nothing else, for the sake of actually listening to someone else. I mean, what good is your point of view? You already know your point of view. If you're going to stick with your point of view, you're going to stay stagnant the rest of your life. The beauty of being able to listen to someone else is to actually expand your point of view and move toward what yogis are concerned with, nonviolence.

What it's trying to do—what this concept of *detachment* is about, really—is allowing you to have points of view, but you just don't berth your ship there. You keep on sailing the ship on the continuum of the present moment. And when you don't have to berth your ship, you don't have to lose the beauty of now because you're stuck in some infatuation with your beliefs.

Another good example is my friend who is a violinist. At seventeen he played at Carnegie Hall. What was he going to do, keep on telling everybody that? "Oh, yeah, at seventeen I played at Carnegie Hall." So his whole life would become this one event, and from then on he would just keep holding on to that one event, so he would never live another moment. Was he not going to live another moment? Was that going to be the peak of his life, and from there on that was all he was going to hold on to? No. He even hates being called a violinist for that reason. Just because he can play the violin, all of a sudden he's identified as a violinist. He hates that.

Hopefully, yoga allows you to stop trying to make yourself significant and important by identifying with beliefs or stories about your past. It's like someone meets you for the first time, and you like them, and you start telling your stories about you, and you sort of become significant in their eyes because you tell them all the things that you've made it through, like, oh, you know, I've made it through a terrible childhood or, oh, no, I was a really privileged kid, I was a special kid. But instead of living in your stories, why not taste the present moment? Isn't it enough? Is it not enough to be alive?

NINA   Well, it's interesting, but I can see that you're still holding on to some things from your past about your body image, your sexuality, and your attractiveness.

ROD   Yes—I'm not saying that I've ascended into some godly level. I'm just saying that yoga practice has seriously aided me in letting go of some of my grip on things that I was obsessive about before.

NINA   How does it do that?

ROD   It's actually simple. I can be very scientific about this if you want.

NINA   Maybe I'll fall asleep while you're talking about science—

ROD   Then the yoga teacher would have accomplished the—

NINA   —impossible.

ROD   —the impossible.

NINA   He's a genius.

ROD   He's a genius! I fell asleep! I took a nap for the first time in my life when he was talking. Oh, God.

NINA   How does it do that wonderful thing?

ROD   How's it do that wonderful thing? It's simple. It rewires you. I already went through it—Pavlov's dog.

NINA   I want to do it. Can I do it?

ROD   The thing that rewires you is your attention to the breath. If you change your breath patterns, you will actually change mental patterns, emotional patterns, and physical patterns. And by working with your attention to your breath, you harness your mind. You learn how to concentrate by paying attention to the direct sensation in the body and bringing your mind back to that sensation. Bring your mind back to the breath—the breath, which is always in the present moment. So by watching your breath, you're accessing the present moment. And when you're in the present moment, you're not in the past or the future. That in itself drastically shifts things.

PART 5

Posing and Reposing

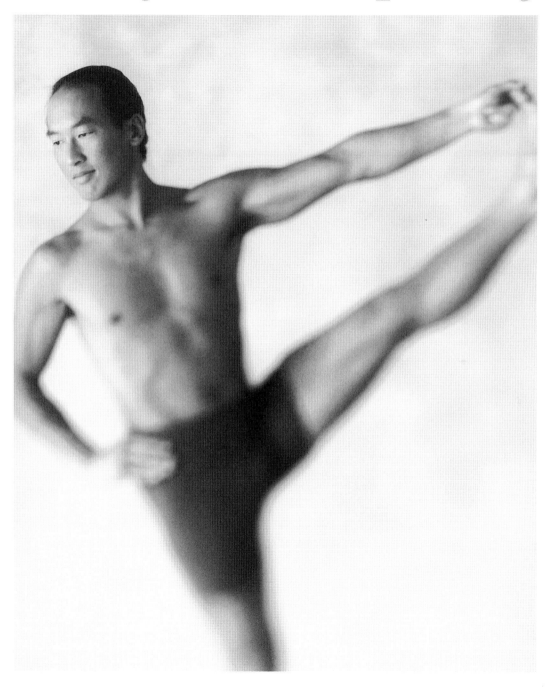

No Word

The trees hang silent
In the heat . . .

Undo your heart
Tell me your thoughts
What you were
And what you are . . .

Like bells no one
Has ever rung.

— KENNETH REXROTH

This part of our book presents detailed photographs and information about a small subset of the thousands of poses that make up yoga. Rodney chose these poses because he considers them to be the basic building blocks for a yoga practice. These basic poses are accessible to everyone, and yet they continue to be unfathomable in their subtleties. As you learn them they can lead you to more difficult poses, and yet on their own they contain all the elements of a complete yoga practice.

Rodney himself still practices all the poses in this book, and we hope that you, too, will return to them again and again. For they are like beautiful simple piano pieces, which although written for beginners, to introduce the structure and concepts of music, are so rich they can be played with deep appreciation by musicians of any skill level.

If you want to learn more about some of the more advanced yoga poses, you can consult one of the books or videos recommended in Appendix A or begin attending yoga classes in your community. Realize, however, that you only need to go into other poses out of a sense of curiosity and fun. Most of the advanced poses just expose and elaborate on movements you can find in the basic poses we have included here.

We are calling this section Posing and Reposing because we feel that doing the yoga postures entails observation and action. *Posing* is when you are observing and listening to the pose. *Reposing* is when you are changing and playing with the pose.

About the Descriptions of the Poses

For each pose in the book, we provide the most basic information about how to get into and explore the pose. We could have gone on and on about alignment subtleties and internal sensations, but instead we have chosen to describe just the foundation movements, from which you can expand on your own. Be playful. Be experimental. Be curious about the feeling, the alignment, the breath, and the movement in each of these poses. For yoga poses are alive in your dialogue with them, not in their perfection. Read the instructions once and periodically reread them whenever you are curious. Look at the photographs again and again to find answers to questions or to raise more questions. Then let yourself be guided by whatever arises naturally. Trust yourself, and let your practice grow intuitively and organically.

About Right and Left

The descriptions for all asymmetrical poses (poses that you do on two sides) are written for the right side only. To do the pose on the left side, simply substitute the word *left* for *right,* and vice versa.

Always do asymmetrical poses on both the right and left sides, starting with the right side first. Time the poses, either by the number of breaths or the number of seconds, so that you spend approximately the same amount of time on the right and left sides.

About Pain

If there is pain in a pose, be curious. Let it be your teacher, not just something you need to endure or avoid. Pain is part of our everyday life—physical pain, emotional pain, and intellectual conflict. If we learn to accept it and feel it, we can begin to integrate it into our lives instead of having it be the catalyst for excessive struggle.

If you feel a strong pain in a pose, try shifting within the pose (backing up from it, moving toward it, walking around it, or going inside it) to see which movements bring deeper understanding of the pain. By shifting inside the pose, you build new patterns of coordination that will allow you to move with ease and harmony. Many of us try to avoid pain because we're scared of hurting ourselves even more, but it is often this avoidance that causes a downward spiraling toward other difficulties in our postures and in our lives.

On the physical level, the more you allow yourself to play with pain, the more you'll understand different qualities of pain. Some pains are definitely more injurious, and some are actual openings. Experience and familiarity will enable you to make this distinction with more and more refinement.

Building a Practice

We organized this part of our book, Posing and Reposing, as a complete yoga practice, sequenced in a manner that arises in the body.

- We start with preparatory poses that give you time to let your mind settle into the movements of your breath and body. They also gently oil all your joints and awaken all your muscles.
- The standing poses come next because they are grounding poses, and they warm up and open your legs, which help you support and access the rest of your body.
- Twists follow the standing poses because they open the outside of your hips, release your groins, and stimulate your internal organs. They also bring awareness and movement to your spine to prepare you for back bends.
- The activity and awareness of standing poses and twists lead into back bends, some of the most vigorous and demanding poses in yoga. Back bends create vulnerability as they open your neck, shoulders, heart, belly, and pelvis.

- We then take the vitality and vulnerability of the back bends into the cooling, centering movements of the seated poses. These seated poses are the neutral poses between the back bends and the forward bends.
- The forward bends soothe your nervous system and turn you inward, preparing you for the quiet, meditative restorative poses.
- The restorative poses conclude the practice, taking you into the observation of your subtle body and allowing you to integrate all that has happened within your practice. End every yoga practice with a restorative pose.

If you wish, you can do all the poses in all of the sections, from preparatory poses to restorative poses, as one long yoga practice, in the order in which they are presented. You can also design your own yoga practice by selecting a subset of the poses from the chapters and then doing just those poses, in the order in which they are presented.

Preparatory Poses

The poses in this section are all good for starting your yoga practice. They enable you to check in with your entire body and bring your awareness to areas that feel discordant, stiff, or just plain yucky at the beginning of a personal practice.

They give your mind time to begin to settle into the present moment, leaving behind your agenda for the day or the residue from the recent past. They are simple poses that derive their integrity from your playfulness and your listening to whatever inner movements are arising.

moving onto your hands and feet
feeling the prowess of your body
undulating your spine

Relax into your back body and let your mind move inward. Fall into the ground. Exhale com-pletely. Fall inward. Become sensitive to the movements and feelings inside. Your body will lead your mind in the dance.

You can also do the poses in this section in the sequence in which they are presented as a short Playful Practice. Be gentle. Delve inward.

Some questions to ask yourself while doing these poses:

- How am I feeling (energetic, lethargic, sad, joyous, relaxed, agitated, introverted, extroverted, silly, angry)?
- How do I feel like moving (fast or slow, dynamically or softly, lyrically or sharply)?
- What is the state of my breath (choppy or smooth, long or short, deep or shallow)?

Happy Baby Pose

30 seconds to 1 minute

DIRECTION OF MOVEMENT

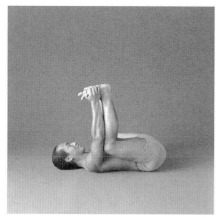

Lie on your back and hold the outsides of your feet with your hands. Let your back body feel broad and long on the ground. As you release inside your hip sockets, feel your sacrum unfurl back toward the ground. The dominant movement should be your spine falling onto the earth, while the pull of your legs is the secondary force. *Surrender.*

Can you feel your spine undulating—from your tailbone to the base of your skull—with the rise and fall of your breath?

ALTERNATE VIEW

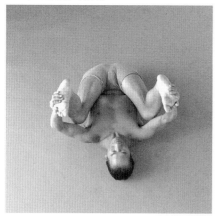

Keep your feet directly over your knees, and let them be awake and vibrant. And keep your chest broad, with your arms drawing down into the support of your heart. Untether your neck and throat from the pull of your legs.

Play. Move your legs. Roll around on your spine. Laugh, even.

MODIFICATION

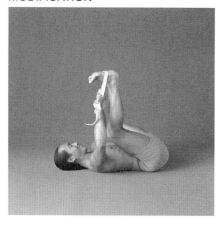

This modification is for people who cannot reach their feet without distorting their spines and shoulder girdles. Using a strap allows you to pay more attention to the opening in your hip sockets and enables you to move your spine naturally and to breathe easily.

When your hips are tight, your body compensates by shortening and jamming your spine, causing retraction (like a roly-poly bug that you've poked with your finger). When you use the strap, you will start feeling that wonderful languid ease that comes from having your back on the ground.

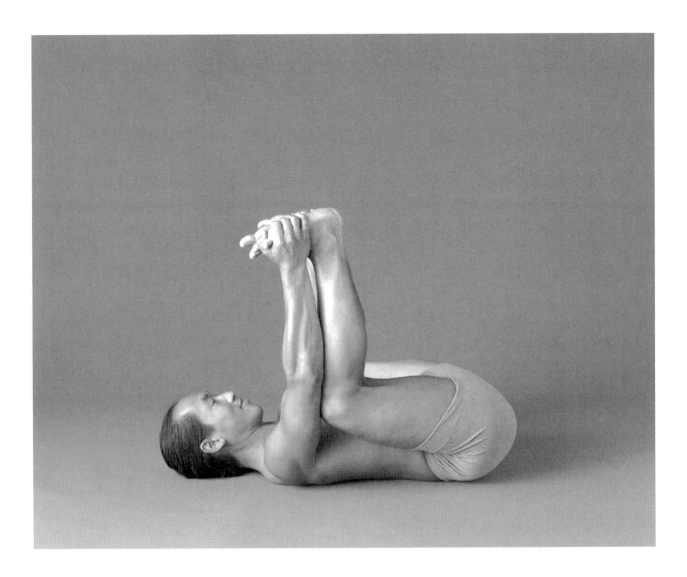

One Thing. The delight of a happy six-month-old baby rolling around on its back and playing with its feet.

Fall in love with suppleness.

Reclined Twist

Jathara Parivartanasana (modified) / 30 seconds to 1 minute

DIRECTION OF MOVEMENT

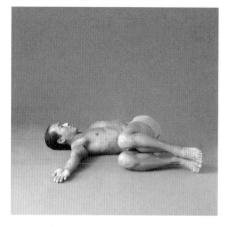

Start by lying on your back with your legs bent, your feet on the ground, and your arms out to the side. Next flex your feet and draw your legs into your chest. Feel your exhalation drop your back body deeply into the ground, your belly receding into the cavity of your pelvis.

On an exhalation, release your legs to the left and bring them to the ground, keeping their vitality as you drop their weight to the earth. Feel how your feet and legs energize your spine and how the length of your spine is like a flower's stem extending into the blossoming of your chest. Lightly extend and press your arms along and into the ground, maintaining the softness of your neck and enhancing the openness of your chest.

ALTERNATE VIEW

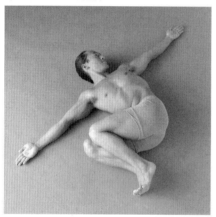

Feel the length of your groins and the natural curve in your lower back. Broaden your chest into the reach of your arms as you keep your neck and throat soft. Breathe into your pelvis, and exhale through your upper chest. Keep your sense organs relaxed and dropping deeply toward the center of your skull.

As the twist continues, feel the length of your spine on the inhalation and the depth of the twist on your exhalation. Inhale down into your pelvis to lengthen and arch your lower back. Exhale into the unwinding and broadness of your back and your chest.

MODIFICATION

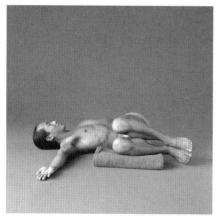

If this twist seems too severe, place a block or folded blanket under your knees and rest them on that lift. Often in twists your breath becomes shallow. This modification will allow your chest to turn enough so your arms can reach along the ground without restriction. It will also allow your breath to run more fully and create waves of motion in your spine.

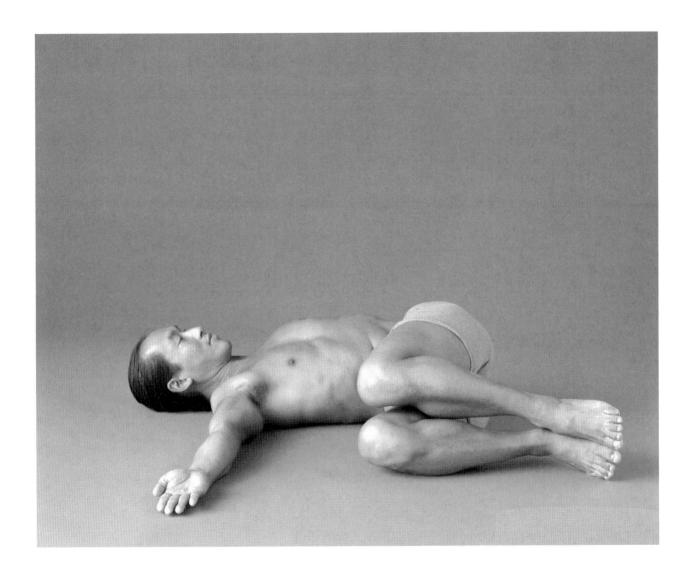

One Thing. Our bodies love to be squeezed and then released, and this twist is like a long, slow squeeze. So as you come back out of the twist, allow yourself to luxuriate in the release.

Let your breath be the thread that weaves your mind and body together.

Reclined Leg Stretch

Supta Padangushthasana / 30 seconds to 1 minute

PREPARATION

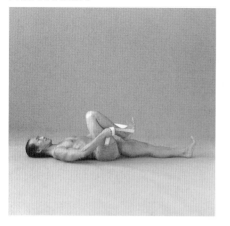

Start by lying on the ground with your legs together, and extend both legs strongly through your heels and into the ground. Feel your side waist lengthen from those roots. Keep your left leg burrowing into the ground as you bend your right leg into your chest. Hold your right big toe with your right hand or—for most people—place a strap around the arch of your right foot. Then extend your right leg straight up from the power of your bottom leg. Maintain the natural curves of your spine as you feel its length from the grounding of your legs. Keep your neck supple, and make sure you are not throwing your head back.

DIRECTION OF MOVEMENT

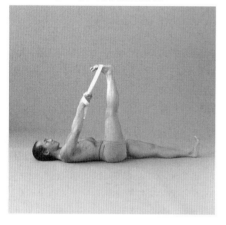

Lengthen and spread your body along the ground. Feel the weight of your raised leg falling back into your hip socket as you reach into the full expression of your foot and length of your bones—from your hip through your knee to your heel. Draw your arms back into the sockets to support the breadth of your chest and the lift of your collarbones.

Inhale into the width of your back body. Exhale into the length of your spine. Try not to be overly enthusiastic about pulling your leg toward your chest. Instead emphasize the grounding of your bottom leg and the equanimity of your mind in the pose as a whole.

MODIFICATION

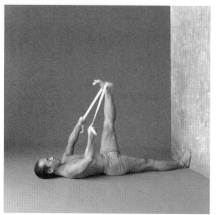

Many of us get lost in the dance of the raised leg. Pressing your foot against a wall will remind you of your foundation (from which your leg of action is moving). Do this modification periodically, alternating your legs as shown here, to remind yourself that this pose—like all poses—is built from the ground up.

Connect—reconnect—again and again to the earth.

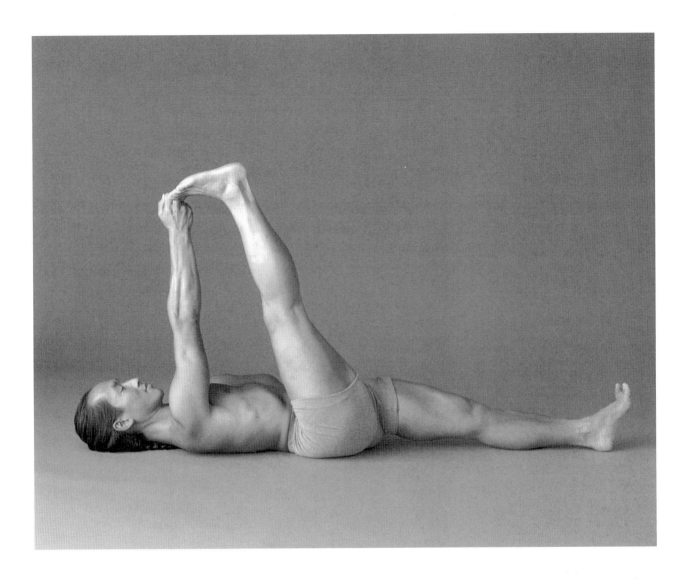

One Thing. Find the vast field of your back body, from which the action of your body can spring forth.

Go into a dream state, yet feel your body even more completely.

Passive Back Bend

Matsyasana (modified) / 1 to 3 minutes

DIRECTION OF MOVEMENT

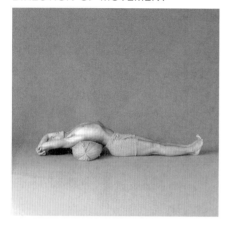

With your shoulder blades placed at the apex of a bolster or blanket roll, extend your legs straight and reach your arms overhead. Then broaden your shoulder blades and move them down your back.

Breathe into the expansion of your back ribs on the bolster and feel how your breath rises into the expansion of your front ribs. Let your spine luxuriate over the curve of the bolster, sensing its length and fluidity. Feel your back muscles broaden out from your spine as they lend support for the back bend.

What is the relationship between your vulnerability and your aliveness?

MODIFICATION

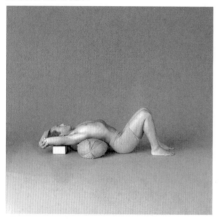

If your head and neck feel uncomfortable being thrown back, place a block, folded blanket, or pillow underneath your head. Adjust the height of the lift under your head so your neck has the same arc as the rest of your spine. Every vertebra should be equal in its responsibility for supporting the shape and weight of your body.

If there is any strain in your lower back, bend your legs and place the soles of your feet on the ground. This will allow you to maintain the natural sway of your back. Feel the continuous, even arc from your tailbone to the crown of your head.

ALTERNATIVE VIEW OF MODIFICATION

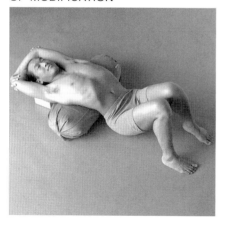

Notice the placement of the bolster in this photograph. Feel free to shift its placement to bring understanding to different parts of your spine, but realize that for most of us it is important to open the upper chest by placing the bolster as shown. Allow the bolster not only to open your chest but also to bring awareness to the breath in your back body.

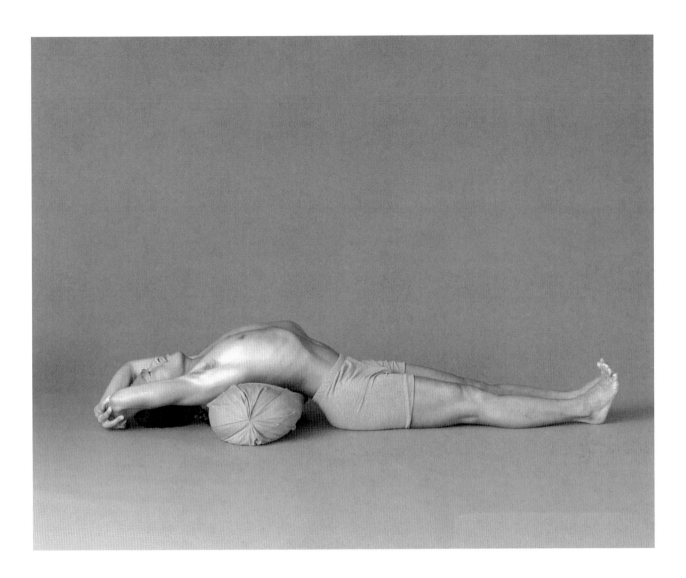

One Thing. Make a sky out of your chest—feel the clear blue of it.

Your body is water, so let the dams open and the water run the riverbed.

Cat Pose

Chakravakasana / 3 to 10 repetitions, with your breath

NEUTRAL

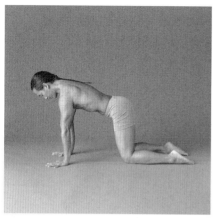

Supported by your arms and legs, feel like a four-legged animal with the weight of your torso and the prowess of your spine supported by your hands and feet. Lengthen your back body toward your tailbone. Extend your front body toward your head. Keep the crown of your head in line with the rest of your spine.

Can you feel as though every vertebra is floating like a cloud on the buoyancy of your breath? Make minute, integrated undulations in your entire spine.

PURRING CAT

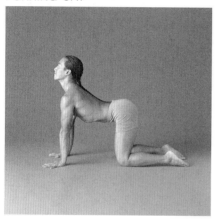

As your shins press downward, lengthen and deepen your groins to raise your sitting bones. From the movement of your groins, your lower back arches into a back bend. Extend your armpit-chest forward and up into the movement of your neck and head arching skyward.

Press your hands into the ground to support your broad, lifting chest. Let the strength of the pose come from your arms and legs as the muscles of your back feel like the broad hood of a cobra. Continue to initiate the arch from your pelvis.

ANGRY CAT

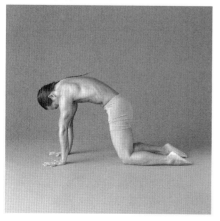

With your hands and feet pressing, drop your tailbone between your legs as your belly hollows. Curl your head downward and back toward your tailbone, and expand your back body. Press your arms downward into the ground to draw your wide, hollow chest into the broadness of your back.

As you inhale, your back body should inflate from the inside out. As you exhale through your nose, your exhalation should feel extended and channeled, like the hissing of a cat.

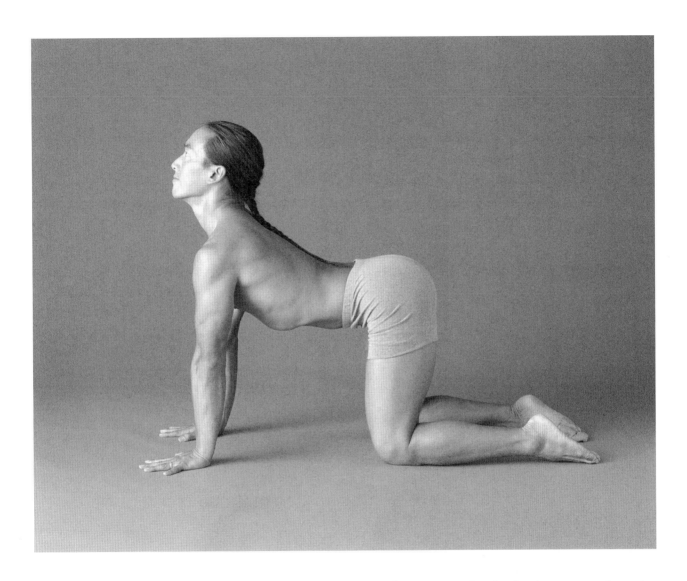

One Thing. Initiate the arching and hunching of your spine from your pelvis, letting it resonate along the entire length of your spine. Observe its rippling effect.

What is gracefulness? The coordination of the breath, the movement of the body, and the observation of the mind.

Downward-Facing Dog

Adho Mukha Shvanasana / 15 seconds to 1 minute

PREPARATION

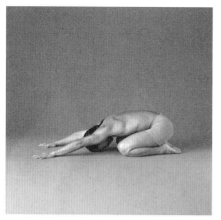

Start in Child's Pose (page 296). Now reach your arms as far forward as possible, keeping them shoulder-width apart. While maintaining this distance between your hands and feet, come to all fours, moving your feet hips-width apart. Then turn your toes under and straighten your legs into Downward-Facing Dog.

Extend and open your shoulders until there is a straight line between your fingertips and your sitting bones.

DIRECTION OF MOVEMENT

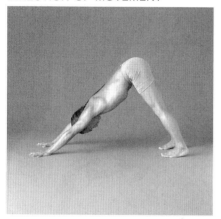

Pull your thighbones back into your hamstrings to elongate your waist, and move into the full extension of your arms. As your heels move toward or into the ground, lift your sitting bones and expand and breathe in your back lower ribs. Search each hand and foot for evenness of contact with the floor, shifting your body weight more and more into center. The more your body is aligned, the more evenly and easily your breath will flow. *The powerful movements of a horse, along with its lightness and grace.*

Soften your temple skin. Soften your brain.

MODIFICATION

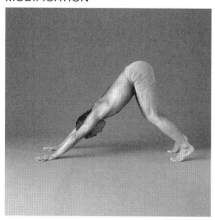

When your hamstrings are tight, your spine is compromised. By bending your legs, you can feel the true length and natural curve of your lower back. This allows your body to fall into a relaxed state from which you can observe more accurately the alignment of your spine.

After bending your knees, play with straightening your legs more and more. This modification is for everybody—it will enable you to understand the relationship between your legs, pelvis, and spine.

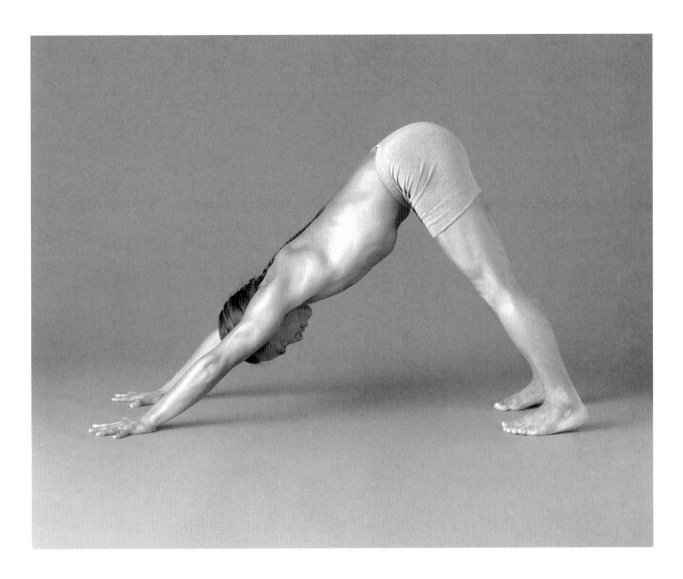

One Thing. We love this pose because it speaks to the totality of our being. Feel the vigor of your arms, the extension of your torso, the power of your legs, and the receptivity of your mind.

Can you find a place where the breath whistles through your body like a beautiful clear note through a flute?

Standing Poses

The poses in this section are good for waking up your legs and arms, opening your hips, and energizing your spine. Energetically they connect you with the earth and center you within yourself.

> *rooting your feet*
> *invigorating your legs*
> *scintillating your spine*
> *singing your arms*

Draw the energy of the earth up from your tactile feet through your powerful legs into your spine. Your spine channels the energy into the emerging opening of your heart and the crown of your head. Your arms and hands become expressions of your feelings and thoughts. Listen to the earth and let it tell you where to walk.

You can do the poses in this section in the sequence in which they are presented as an energizing and awakening practice that will help you move with confidence in the world.

Some questions to ask yourself while doing these poses:

- How even is my weight on my feet?
- Do I feel the connection between my legs and my spine?
- Are my arms helping support and lift my heart?
- Can I move from my feet up instead of from my head down?
- Can I work strongly and surrender at the same time?

Mountain Pose

Tadasana / 15 seconds to 1 minute

DIRECTION OF MOVEMENT

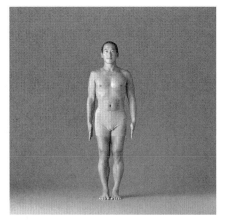

Stand with your feet together. Feel the strength of your legs rooting into the ground—a visceral connection to the earth. Then, as your legs root downward, feel your supple spine rise up. Broaden your back body as you lift your upper chest, expanding your collarbones into the wings of your arms.

Imagine a basket of sweet, ripe mangoes is on your head, and balance it sensuously as you extend up into it. Smell the fragrance of the fruit and let the juice drip down the inside center of your mind and spine. *Length, width, and depth without rigidity.*

ALTERNATE VIEW

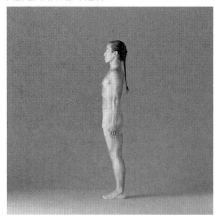

Sense the plumb line of your body, down from the center of your head through the center of your heart through the center of your pelvis to the fronts of your heels. Now feel the natural curves of your spine—a slight back bend in your lower back, a slight roundedness in your upper back, and a slight back bend in your neck.

Then play with your balance. Fall in different directions: fall forward, fall backward, fall sideways, fall into center. Don't assume your habitual posture is centered. *Breathe it, feel it, relax into it, fall into it, rise from it.*

MODIFICATION

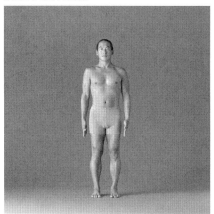

For those of you who are knock-kneed or feel unstable with your feet together, try standing with your feet hips-distance apart and parallel. This will help you feel more grounded.

This modification allows for more stability and more emphasis on broadness and space, and it is good for all of us to do once in a while.

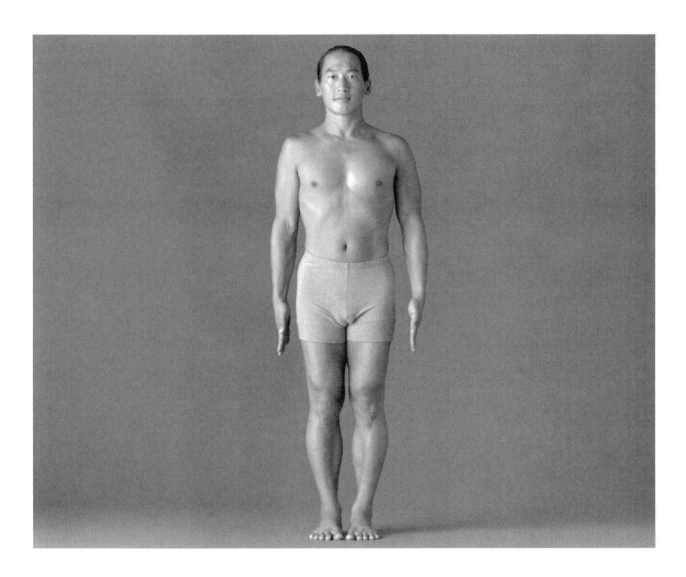

One Thing. An infinite play of movement—an ongoing conversation. What is the center of the center?

falling, retrieving, balancing—
falling, retrieving, balancing—
falling, retrieving, balancing . . .

Volcano Pose

Urdhva Hastasana / 15 seconds to 1 minute

DIRECTION OF MOVEMENT

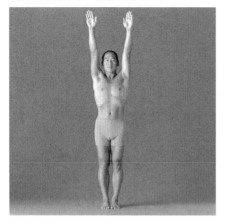

Draw the energy of the earth up through your body and out through your fingertips. As you feel the strong movement of your arms and legs, feel also the length but ease of your spine. Allow your upper chest to support the reach of your arms as your arms help your chest fly upward. Keep your neck soft and your sense organs receptive. And encourage the tremendous extension of your arms and legs without hardening or locking your joints.

As your arms, legs, and torso are vigorously expanding, let your neck be as supple as a swan's.

ALTERNATE VIEW

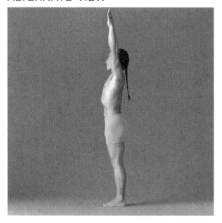

Open your body naturally into a slight back bend, keeping your breastbone receptive and open. As your shoulder blades press firmly against your back, take your upper arms farther and farther behind your ears. Keep your side waist elongated from the depth of your groins to the length of your armpits, but feel the even suspension of your ribs as your arms spray upward, like the steam that rises when lava meets the ocean.

The strength of your legs and the exhaltation of your arms uplift the energy of your heart.

MODIFICATION

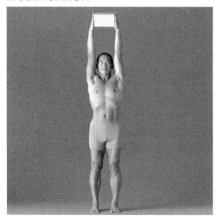

Place a block between your hands and extend it skyward. Feel your entire body, from your feet to the block, inching its way to its full length. As you continue to extend, maximize the wideness of the muscles of your back away from your spine.

Sometimes using extra weight in a pose—like this block in Volcano Pose—helps us break postural habits by increasing the feedback from our bodies to our minds.

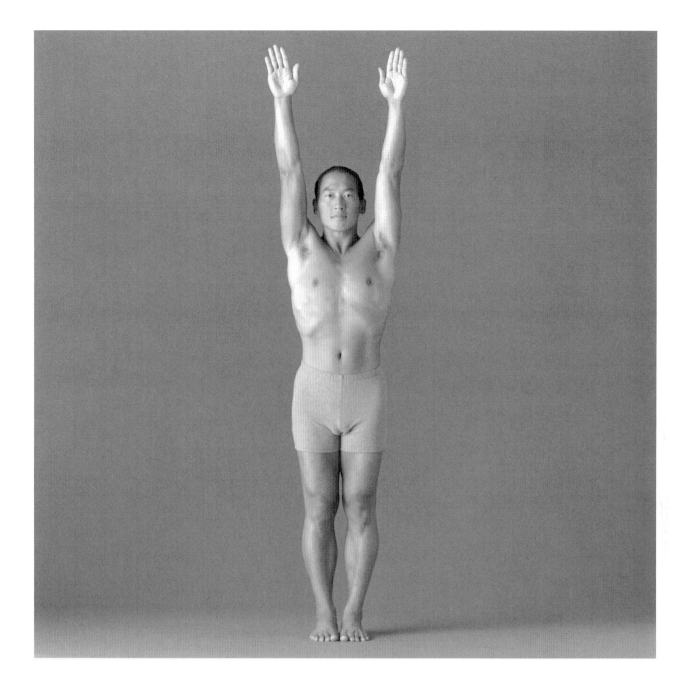

One Thing. Feet connected to the mind, mind connected to the feet. Raising the earth to the heavens.

Don't let your neck be the noose of your orientation. Don't strangle yourself just to let yourself feel alive.

Standing Forward Bend

Uttanasana / 10 seconds to 1 minute

DIRECTION OF MOVEMENT

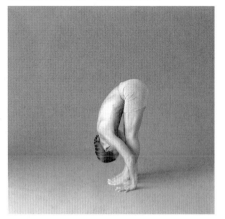

As you deepen and drop your groins backward, fold your pelvis over your thighs and cascade your spine over the earth of your legs. As your feet plant themselves, let your legs draw energy up from the earth like the vibrant trunk of a tree. *Pelvis liquid, spine flowing, neck and head giving.*

Breathe into the broadness of your hamstrings. Then search for balance between front and back, teetering from the fulcrum at the fronts of your heels.

MODIFICATION 1

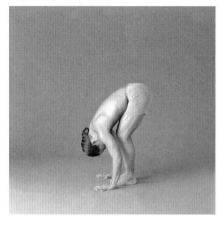

This modification is for those who have tight hamstrings. It allows the folding to take place at your hip sockets instead of in your lower back. It also increases the surrender of your spine.

Bend your legs enough so that any tension in your back is released. Let your body be supported by your thighs. Spread your toes, and ground your heels.

Allow the bending of your legs to help you focus on the folding at your hip creases. On your exhalation, let your breath drop completely out of your body.

MODIFICATION 2

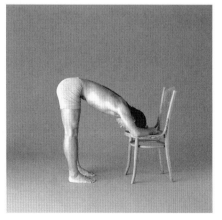

This modification is a restorative pose. When you rest the weight of your head, your nervous system cools down. This modification also relieves your spine and keeps it from taking too much pull from the weight of your upper body and your head.

Be sure to pick the appropriate height for your prop (a block or a chair) so you can easily rest the area between your forehead and the crown of your head on it.

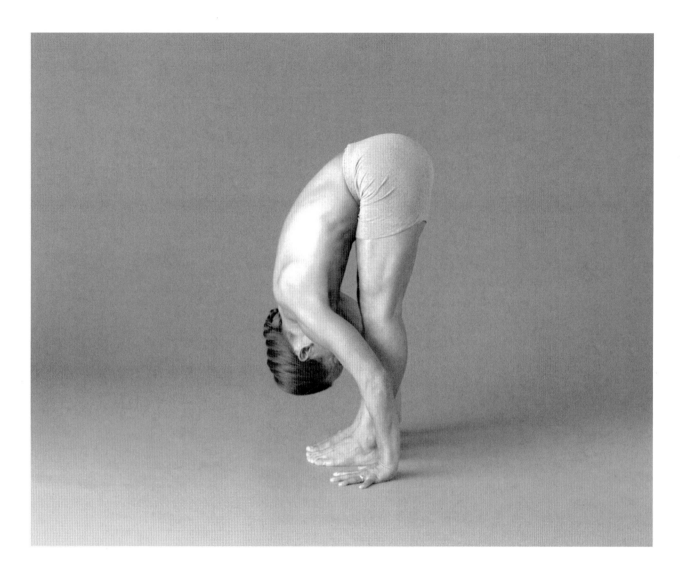

One Thing. From the sturdiness of the legs flows the liquid spine.

What is it not to understand intellectually but to be so neutral that the listener becomes the sound?

Extended Standing Forward Bend

Uttanasana 2 / 5 to 20 seconds

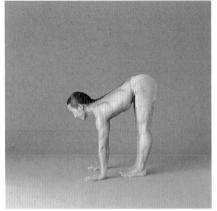

From Standing Forward Bend (page 234), drop the top of your sacrum and lower back into a back bend as you arc your spine into the forward lifting of your chest and head. Don't strain your neck—lift your head only to the point where the arch in your neck is congruous with the arch in the rest of your spine. Coming onto your fingertips, reach your arms into the ground to further support the opening of your heart and the expansion of your lungs. Use your arms and legs as the source of power to extend and support your spine.

Activate the arches of your feet strongly, and from the grounding of your fingertips lift the dome of your hands—your entire body lit up.

MODIFICATION 1

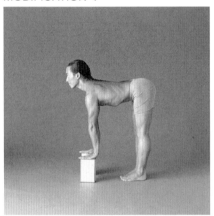

If you can't reach the ground or your back has to round to do so, place your hands on blocks, pressing down as your chest extends forward. Make sure not to jam your knees; draw up the fronts of your thighs so that your kneecaps are lifted. Come down only as far as you can while keeping your lower back in a slight back bend.

Feel that the main movement is the folding of your pelvis over your legs and the supple reach of your spine. Inhale into your pelvis. Exhale into the length of your spine.

MODIFICATION 2

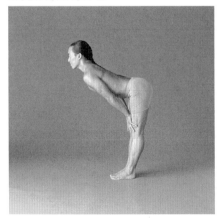

If you can't reach the ground or your back has to round to do so, place your hands on the tops of your thighs, pressing back as your chest extends forward. Spread your toes, plant your heels, draw up your legs strongly, and arc your spine. Keep your chest broad, with your arms fully expanded. Let your heart and lungs be supple while your sternum and ribs stay soft. *Chest moving forward as groins move back.*

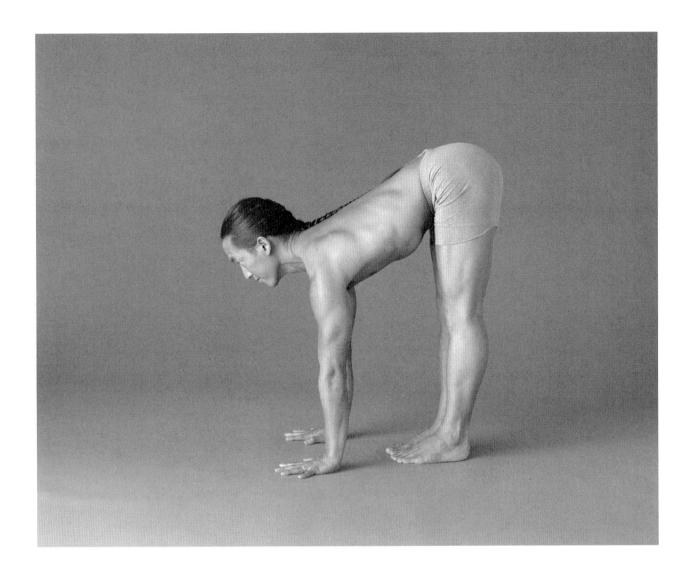

One Thing. The spine surging forth from the anchor of the legs.

Don't define yourself by pushing yourself to feel the stretch. Instead, go into the emptiness—the void from which your life is streaming out.

Lunge

5 to 20 seconds

DIRECTION OF MOVEMENT

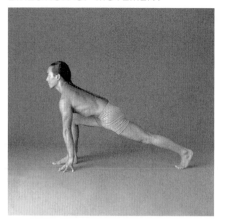

Keep your back leg straight and extending strongly through your heel while your front leg is bent to 90 degrees (the front shin perpendicular and thigh parallel to the ground). Come up to your fingertips and elongate the front of your spine, from the release of your groins back to the forward movement of your collarbones. Gaze forward. Press both feet firmly into the ground, and extend your spine from that foundation. Feel the dynamic opposition between the movements of your two legs.

Can you maintain fluidity in your hip sockets and extend your spine without making it rigid? Inhale into the extension of your back leg. Exhale into the elongation of your spine.

ALTERNATE VIEW

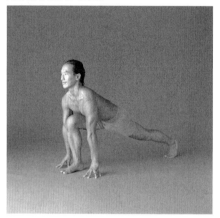

Keep your front knee moving in the same direction as your third toe. Spread your toes, and extend the soles of your feet. Bring your awareness to the tactile sensations of your fingertips and your feet on the earth. Let your legs carry the weight of your body as your hands lightly touch the floor and guide the opening of your heart.

Feel the springiness of your legs and the buoyancy of your heart and lungs.

MODIFICATION

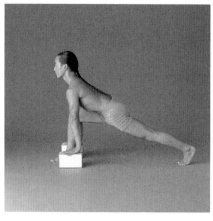

If your hips are tight and your back leg does not extend easily while your front leg is at 90 degrees, place your hands on blocks to bring your spine closer to its natural curves and, if needed, unbend your front leg until there is a sense of rising up from the earth.

Your spine should feel as if it is riding on and rising up from the platform of your legs and feet. So straighten your front leg to the point where your torso feels supported by it and not dragged down by it. Deepen your front thigh toward the ground while your back leg lifts up toward the ceiling. This dynamic grounding and opposition of your legs will cause an upwelling of energy in your torso.

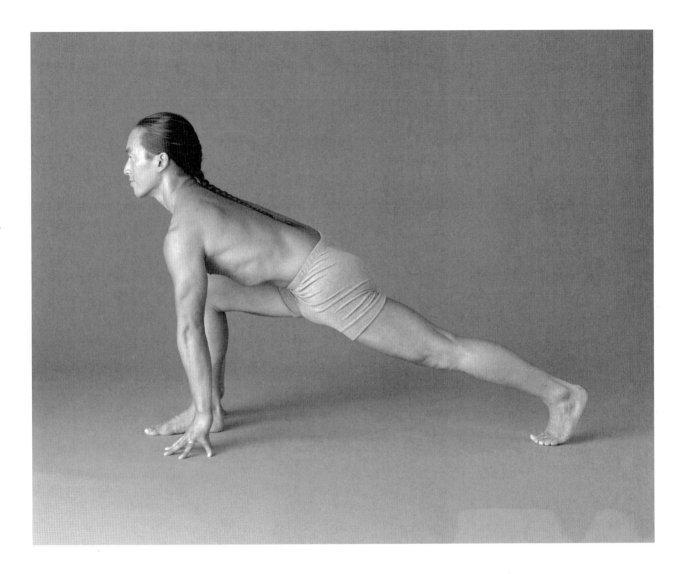

One Thing. From the Roman columns of your legs, look forward with your heart.

It's not your brain that lifts you, it's your legs that lift you.

Triangle Pose

Trikonasana / 15 to 45 seconds

PREPARATION

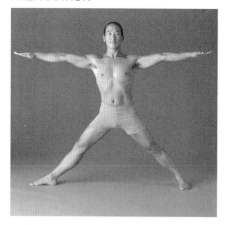

Extend your arms out to the side and then take a wide stride, so your feet are directly under your fingertips. Turn your left foot slightly in. Next turn your right foot out completely so that your big toe points directly to the right. Then, with both your legs drawing up from tenacious feet, extend your spine majestically upward. Feel the broadness of your back body with the lift of your front body.

DIRECTION OF MOVEMENT

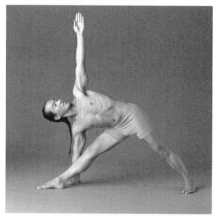

From the earthy strength of your legs, spill your pelvis over your front leg so that the weight of your body is moving into your back heel. And from the constant grounding of your back leg, elongate your spine. Press your bottom arm into the ground, supporting the openness and broadness of your chest into the reach of your top arm. Gaze upward as you soften your core—your throat, your heart, your belly.

Your torso will open up like those kites you made when you were a kid when you strung the crossbar and stretched the soft tissue.

MODIFICATION

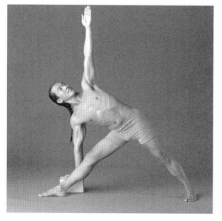

To compensate for tightness in your hamstrings and allow the extension of your spine, especially on the bottom side, place your bottom hand on a prop. Instead of leaning on the block, press into it as you lift your torso from the strength of your bottom arm. Remember that you are trying to open your heart and support your core being with the movement and action of your arms and legs. This modification enables you to achieve freedom of breath and general ease and observation. It also helps you keep the integrity of your back leg—its contact and rootedness to the earth. *Your back leg and foot are the foundation. Your front leg and your arms dance.*

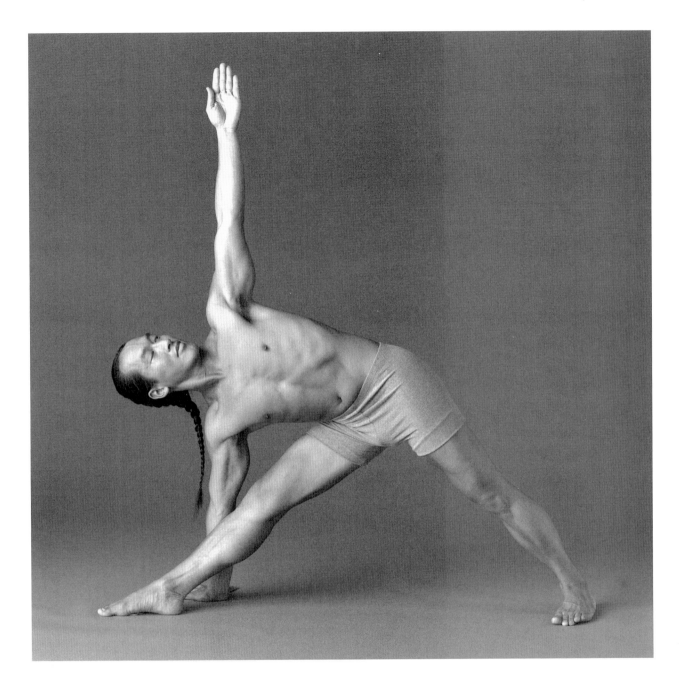

One Thing. Feel how the triangular foundation of your legs generates energy up through your spine and out through the spreading wings of your arms.

Feel the shape of the pose—
breathe it
digest it
play with it

Side Angle Pose

Utthita Parshvakonasana / 10 to 30 seconds

PREPARATION

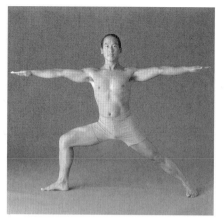

Extend your arms out to the side and then take a wide stride, so your feet are directly under your fingertips. Turn your left foot slightly in. Next, turn your right foot out completely so that your big toe points directly to the right. Then, with both your legs drawing up from broad extended feet, bend your front leg to 90 degrees, bringing your shinbone perpendicular to the ground, right over your ankle. Exhale and bring your right fingertips to the ground, and fully extend your left arm beside your right ear.

DIRECTION OF MOVEMENT

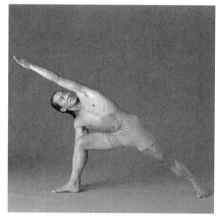

Ground your pelvis in the direction of your back leg as you elongate your bottom waist with the reach of your top arm. Dig your heels deeply as you launch your chest from your pelvis, and rotate both knees away from each other (external rotation). Use your bottom arm to support and broaden your upper chest while you continue to align your skeleton from your back heel through the fingertips of your top hand. Feel your body spiraling from the earth to the sky, unfurling the strength of your legs into a torso filled with light. *Youthful arms bursting forth—reaching for the sun.*

MODIFICATION

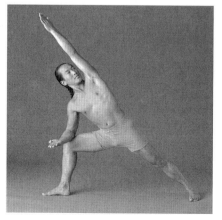

This modification reminds you that the direction of movement for your spine is up from your legs, not down toward the ground. When your hips feel tight, putting your elbow on your knee instead of putting your hand to the ground allows your hips to become an open channel through which energy can move easily from your legs to your spine. This frees up your breath and allows your heart and lungs to be supported, not compromised.

You should use this modification if bringing your hand to the ground creates any contortion of your spine, holding of your breath, or unevenness of your feet. This is often a very congested and frustrating pose, so back up until you have a sense of ease.

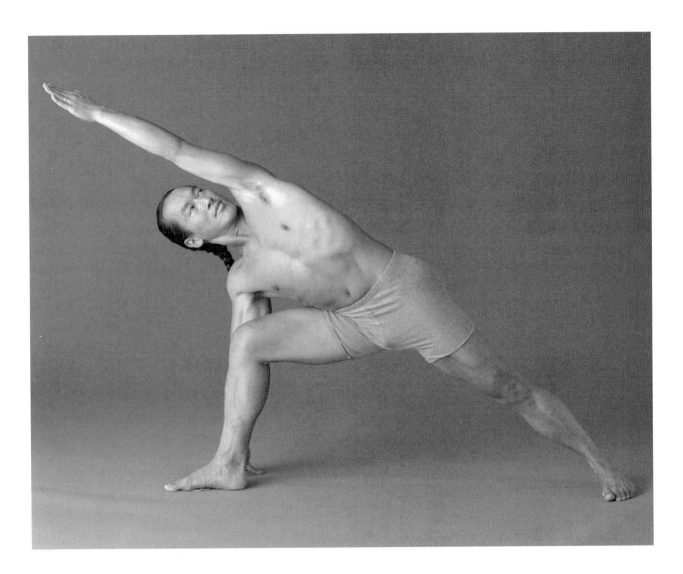

One Thing. Know that even in the midst of difficulty, there is wide open sky. Blue lupines, wild irises, California poppies.

I'm not asking you to work harder, I'm asking you to work differently.

Tree Pose

Vrkshasana / 15 to 30 seconds

PREPARATION

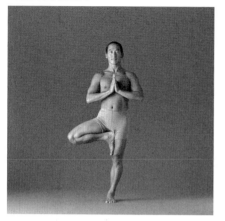

Standing in Mountain Pose (page 230), draw your right heel up to your left inner thigh. Place your palms together in *namaste*, as shown in the photograph.

Be playful with center as you rise up through your core. Let your bent leg feel like a heavy tree branch releasing out from your hip. Continue to sway with the rise and fall of your breath as you steady your mind on the observation of these gentle movements. Feel how your feet and ankles articulate with the ground. *The center of your sternum and your lower ribs like the soft feathers of a bird's chest.*

DIRECTION OF MOVEMENT

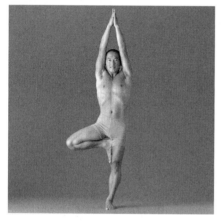

Press down into both heel bones and rise up from the arches of your feet into the base of your pelvis, feeding the reach of your arms over your head. Feel as though your entire outer body has the aliveness of a tree, with nutrients flowing on the surface and a core that is quiet and steady. Let your breath pour into your body like light. Let your exhalation rise up and trace the curves of your spine through to the crown of your head.

Feel a deep, soothing quality, as if your nervous system were bathed in warm sunlight.

MODIFICATION

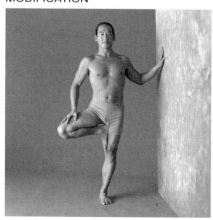

With your feet in Mountain Pose, place your left hand against a wall with your arm slightly bent. Then draw your right leg up into Tree Pose. Use the wall to steady yourself so you can play around with the alignment of this pose. Then reach your right arm up above your head. When you feel balanced, take your left arm up, too. Keep using the wall to catch yourself as you fall off balance—this allows you to be a little more free in your experiments with center.

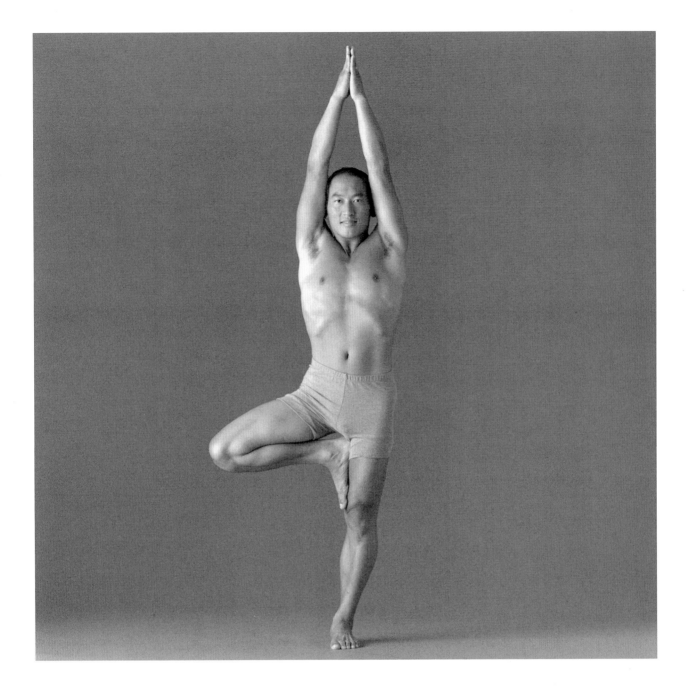

One Thing. Allowing yourself to sway, to pause, and sometimes to fall is the essence of the aliveness of Tree Pose.

Don't assume that the movement you're doing is the movement that's bringing you into balance.

Warrior Pose 1

Virabhadrasana 1 / 15 to 30 seconds

PREPARATION 1

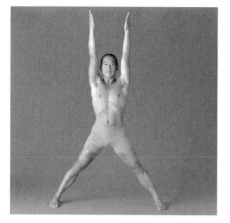

Extend your arms out to the side and then take a wide stride, so your feet are directly under your fingertips. With your feet parallel, raise your arms over your head. Elongate through your waist, from the grounding of your legs to the reach of your arms. Firm your back body toward your front body as you maintain the broadness of your sacrum and shoulder blades. Keep your neck soft and your eyes relaxed.

PREPARATION 2

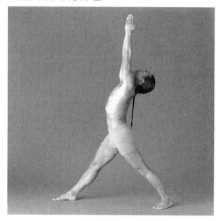

From parallel feet, pivot on your left heel and turn your left foot in 45 degrees, then pivot on your right heel and turn your right foot out to 90 degrees. Inhale, extending vigorously into the reach of your arms. Then turn your pelvis and your chest to the right to face the direction of your right leg.

Feel the broad connection of your feet to the earth, and the earth's energy surging upward into the vibrancy of your legs and spiraling into the height of your spine.

DIRECTION OF MOVEMENT

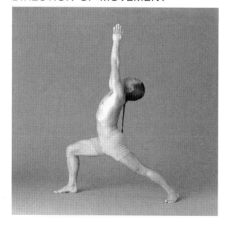

Bend your right leg either toward or all the way to 90 degrees while maintaining the continual grounding of your back heel. Feel your spine emerging from your back leg into a graceful arch. Lengthen your lower back by moving your sitting bones and your tailbone down toward the ground as your back lower ribs broaden and rise up with the reach of your arms. Use your arms to support the opening of your heart—the compassion of your heart spreading into your fingertips. *A celebration. A luminous, joyous face.*

Let your arms help liberate you. Fly upward with your arms.

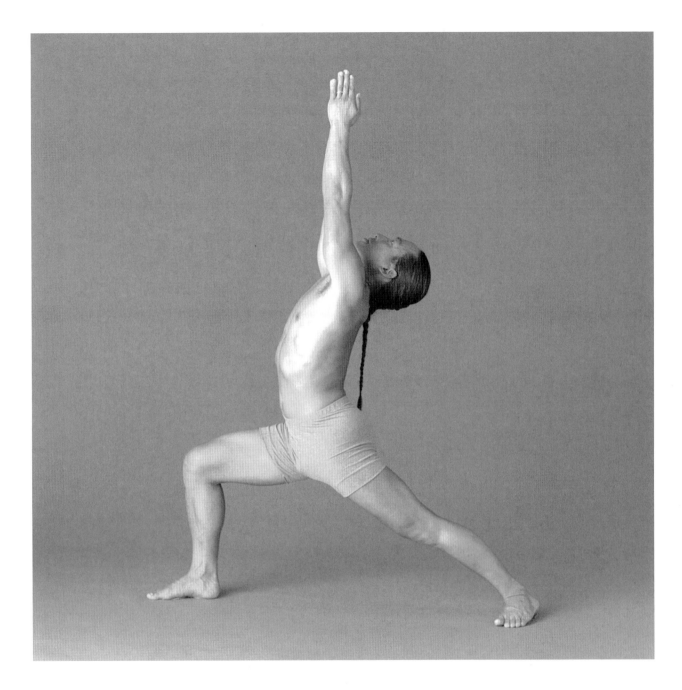

One Thing. A wonderful arc of equanimity, from your heels to your fingertips.

Look into the blue sky and get lost.

Warrior Pose 2

Virabhadrasana 2 / 15 to 30 seconds

PREPARATION

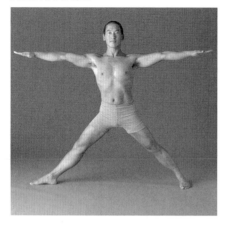

Extend your arms out to the side and then take a wide stride, so your feet are directly under your fingertips. Turn your left foot slightly in. Next turn your right foot out so that your big toe points directly to the right.

Rotate both knees away from each other (external rotation). Reach down into your back (left) outer heel, creating a strength through your back leg—a strength without rigidity. Then pulse your back leg into the earth, and allow the pulsations to build into the expansion of your spine and the reach of your arms.

DIRECTION OF MOVEMENT

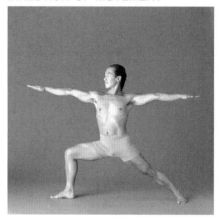

Search for greater contact with your back foot, and from that grounding, bend your right leg to 90 degrees, pressing both outer heels into the ground, and turn your head to look over the middle finger of your right hand. Pump the energy up your legs from the arches of your feet, and let this upward force surge through the gateways of your hips into the unfurling of your spine. Allow the strong reach of your back arm to draw your upper torso over your back leg. This will enable you to support your weight evenly with both legs. Press your shoulder blades into your back, and broaden your collarbones, feeling the sweep from your back arm to your front arm like a single stroke of a Chinese paintbrush.

MODIFICATION

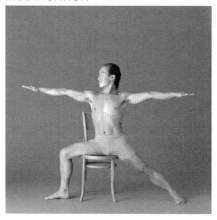

Use this modification to sustain the pose longer and to open your hips more easily. With your weight being carried by the chair, you can play with slightly different positions of your pelvis to discover when the energy of both your legs flows most easily through your pelvis into your spine.

With the seat of the chair underneath you, take a wide stride. Turn your left foot in and your right foot out, and then bend your right knee toward or to 90 degrees. Allow the chair to assist with supporting your weight, but keep your legs as strong as possible.

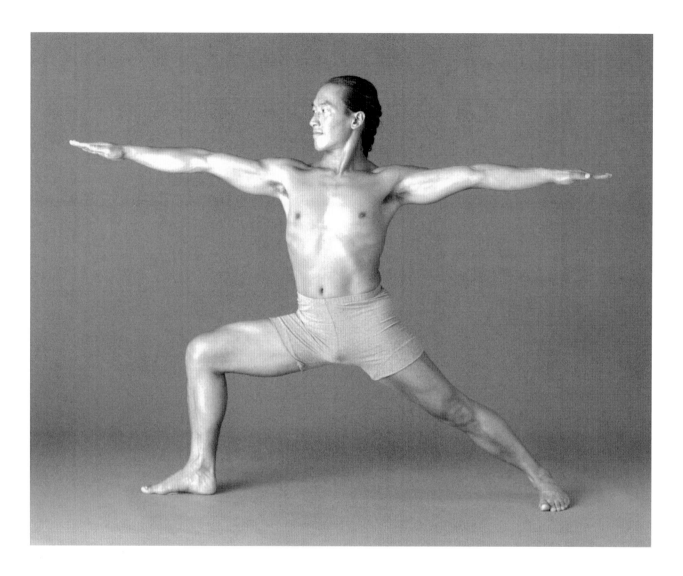

One Thing. Your back leg is your home. So let it be the source of your mindfulness and support.

Stay in the configuration you achieved with struggle, but let go of the struggle. What did you let go?

Half-Moon Pose

Ardha Chandrasana / 15 to 25 seconds

PREPARATION

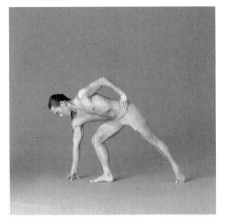

Start in Triangle Pose (page 240). For a few moments, let go of your anticipation and continue to be alive in Triangle Pose. Then, bending your right leg so that your knee aims in the direction of your middle toe, step your back foot toward your front foot and begin to shift your weight onto your front foot, calculating your balance.

Shift your hand about a foot in front of your baby toe as you lift your back leg parallel to the ground. Carefully straighten your supporting leg, feeling as though the weight of your body is right over the thrust of your supporting leg.

DIRECTION OF MOVEMENT

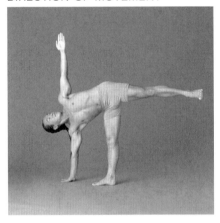

Extend your back leg vigorously and let it be the source of your orientation. The sensitivity and aliveness of your feet give you the necessary feedback to continue to balance. Slowly take your body more and more into one plane, and feel the effortlessness that comes from alignment.

Take off—fly. Your whole body expanding from the pedestal of one foot. Let go of the entanglements of your fear. Broaden your chest from the expanse of the wings of your outstretched arms, riding the winds of your breath. You will have a tendency to be in front of center since there is so much fear of falling backward. Can you creep toward the precipice by leaning your body backward, willing to fall?

MODIFICATION

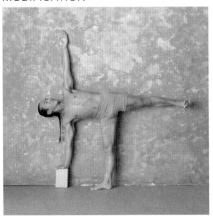

This modification allows you to use the wall as a reference to keep the alignment of your body in the same plane. Since your back heel and your buttocks—and possibly your shoulder blades—will be touching the wall, you can also use the wall to alleviate the fear of falling, which will give you the opportunity to open more freely.

Start in Triangle Pose with your back body and your feet about three inches from the wall. Then move into Half-Moon Pose. If reaching the ground restricts the opening of your chest and the elongation of your spine, use a block under your bottom hand.

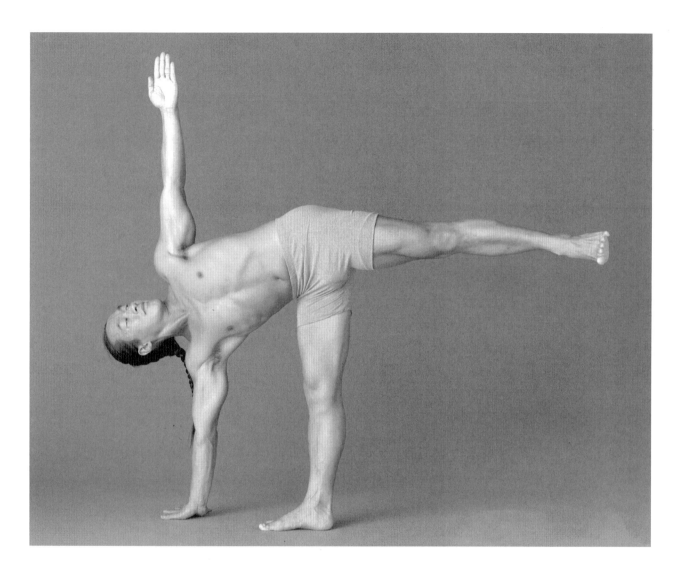

One Thing. You can be so directly on your bones that you can fly. If nothing else, dream it for a moment.

We use most of our energy holding up the illusion of control—it's fictitious—it's tiring.

Sideways Extension Pose

Parshvottanasana / 15 to 30 seconds

PREPARATION

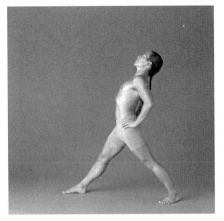

Extend your arms out to the side and then take a wide stride, so your feet are directly under your fingertips. With your feet parallel, place your hands on your hips or take them into *namaste* behind your back. Next, turn your left foot in 45 degrees and your right foot out 90 degrees. Then turn your hips, torso, and head toward the right.

Inhale and bend back over your back leg as your front leg reaches more completely into the splay of your toes. Exhale and guide your pelvis into folding over your front leg. As you are making this movement, continue to ground your pelvis through your back heel. Allow your spine to round as you continue to feel the extension of your front body.

DIRECTION OF MOVEMENT

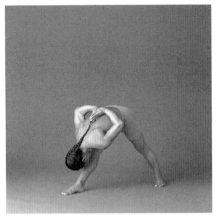

Feel the triangular shape of your legs as they evenly carry the weight of your torso. Let your front body extend to its full length as the forward bending of your spine takes the shape of a crescent moon. Surrender your neck and head completely to the pull of gravity. Draw your elbows slightly up toward the ceiling, firming your shoulder blades into your back but away from your spine to support your supple, open chest, the palace of your heart and lungs. Fully subjugate your mind to the rhythms of your breath and the mountainous strength of your legs.

MODIFICATION

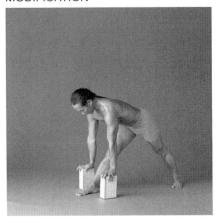

If your hamstrings are not flexible enough, your spine will compensate for the lack of movement in your pelvis, and this may strain your lower back. Therefore you should modify this pose by placing your hands on blocks on either side of your front leg. Feel the length of the front of your spine as well as the forward bending. Observe the ability of your breath to fluctuate from the base of your pelvis to the crown of your head. Don't let your desire to put your head on your shin compromise the equanimity of your breath in this pose.

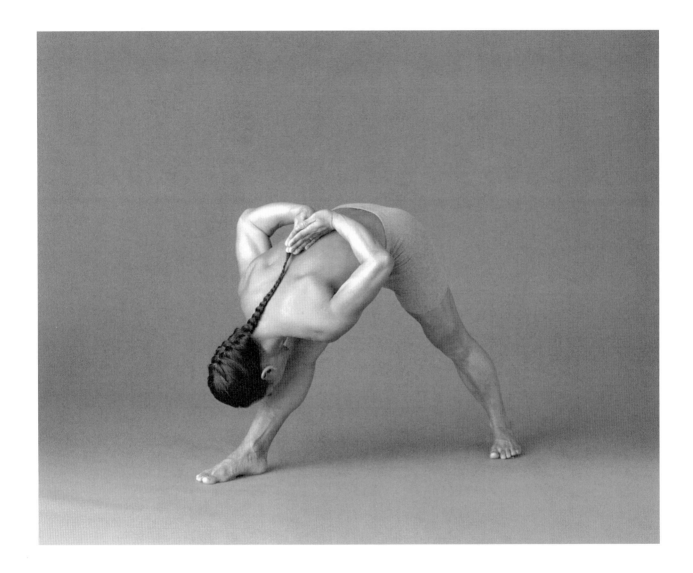

One Thing. The opening of your body will respond to gentleness, attention, and your breath.

If you are pushing too hard, your mental body becomes like a sword instead of a cloud.

Powerful Pose

Utkatasana / 10 to 20 seconds

PREPARATION

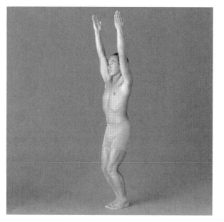

Start in Mountain Pose (page 230). On an inhalation, bend your legs and take your arms over your head. Allow your upper body to slant forward to counterbalance the backward movement of your hips. Reach your arms vigorously upward and back behind your ears. Throughout your movement into the pose, let your legs remain the source of power, and allow the extension of your torso and arms to arise from that power. Feel free to experiment with sitting more deeply into this pose, but don't go so far that you feel any strain in your lower back or shoulders.

DIRECTION OF MOVEMENT

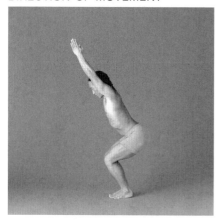

Press your thighs down into your strong, articulate feet as your pelvis is propelled upward into the reach of your arms. Lift your chest both from its connectedness to your arms and from the strength of your legs. Extend the front, back, and sides of your waist evenly. Let your neck be supple, your eyes be receptive, and your throat be clear. Continue to articulate the natural curves of your spine. *Compressed energy springing upward.* Sometimes there is so much vibrancy in our bodies that is being repressed and caged in. One of the translations of the Sanskrit name of this pose is "fierce," so don't be timid about exploring that aspect of it.

MODIFICATION

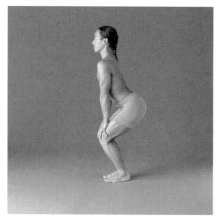

If this pose feels too vigorous or if it irritates your lower back, place your hands on your thighs to give you extra support to lengthen your spine and widen the muscles of your lower back. With your arms below your head, this pose will be much less taxing on your heart and lungs.

With your hands on your knees, you might be able to bend deeper by moving your shinbones forward and your thighbones toward your hamstrings.

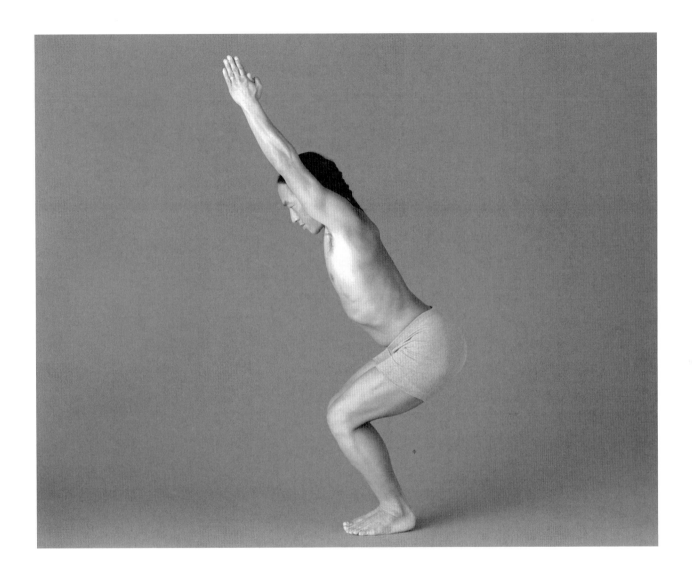

One Thing. Nature sometimes expresses itself fiercely and violently (the eruption of a volcano, the tremor of an earthquake, the surging of a tidal wave). Your body also has this nature—allow yourself to revel in it.

Don't keep your breath in your forehead—let it drop all the way to your groins.

Twists

The poses in this section are good for releasing tension in your spine, breaking open the outer bindings of your hips, and squeezing and releasing the sponge of your body. Twists allow you to be soft, fluid, and organic in your body movements. When you use force in a twist, it reveals how your mind is often directed and determined, reminding you to lead more from your center—your belly—and simply observe with your mind.

> *rising energy from the earth*
> *spiraling spine from the legs*
> *opening chest to the sky*
> *surrendering mind to the breath*

Go inside yourself. Find your breath winding upward, revealing the spiraling nature of your body. Support this nature with your arms, feeling the extension on the inhalation and the turning on the exhalation. Feel the constant give and take, the ebb and flow of the waters of your body.

You can do the poses in this section in the sequence in which they are presented as a revitalizing practice that will tune you into and allow you to move from your center, so no matter what happens, the quietness of your center can be the source of your action and receptivity.

Some questions to ask yourself while doing these poses:

- Am I holding my breath?
- Am I leading with my head?
- Is the spiral of my body even from feet to crown of head?
- Do my heart and my lungs feel supported and opened?

Bharadvaja's Pose

Bharadvajasana / 15 to 30 seconds

PREPARATION

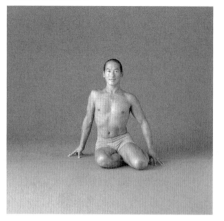

Sitting with your legs in front of you, swing both your feet beside your left hip and place your left ankle in the arch of your right foot, as shown in the photo. Then take your left hand to your right knee as you support yourself with your right hand on the ground. Initiate the twist from your pelvis—don't worry, it's fine if your left hip comes off the ground.

Inhale as you extend your spine. Exhale as you turn to the right.

DIRECTION OF MOVEMENT

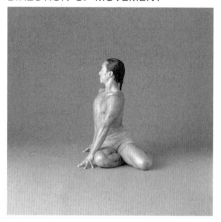

Feel the organic, sensual curves of your hips rising from your joined legs into the spiraling of your spine. Breathe into the sensuality, allowing your inhalation to float your spine up from the mermaid's tail of your legs. Let your exhalation turn you deeper into emptiness, an emptiness that is brought to life through the ease of your body and relaxation of mind.

Feel the airiness and lightness of your chest and the broadness and spaciousness of your back muscles spanning from the center of your spine. Continue to initiate the twist from the ground up, so your neck and head are receptive to the spiral.

MODIFICATION

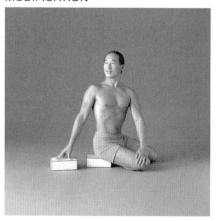

If your pelvis tilts when you sweep your legs around to one side, jamming one side of your waist, sit on a block while doing the twist and have a second block under your right hand so your chest and pelvis stay level. This modification allows your spine to be more level, which allows it to twist more easily. It also gives an ease to your knees, putting less weight and pressure in your knee joints. Many times the congestion in a twist will cause frustration and aggression. The space that is created when you use a lift allows you to enjoy the benefits and cleansing of the twist without the sense of claustrophobia.

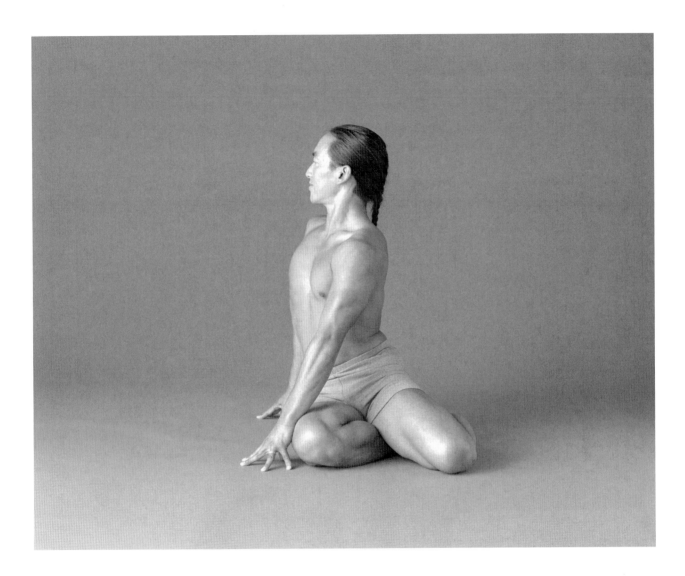

One Thing. Let the easy asymmetry of the foundation of your legs give rise to a sensuous winding and rising of your spine.

The secret is to keep watching—the knots will untie themselves.

Reclined Thigh-Over-Thigh Twist

15 to 45 seconds

PREPARATION

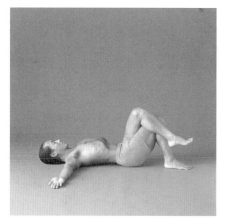

Start by lying on your back with your legs bent and the soles of your feet on the ground. Now cross your right thigh over your left thigh, letting your back body spread on the ground as your belly drops toward your back, as shown in the photo.

Inhale and feel the natural curves of your spine. Then exhale and move your hips four to five inches to the right, and release your legs over to the left. Spiral your spine into the turn of your head to the right.

DIRECTION OF MOVEMENT

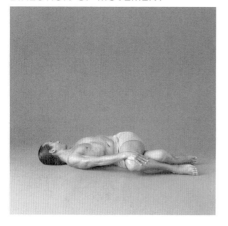

On your inhalation, feel the natural arch of your lower back pulsing open into the expanse of your chest. The outreach of your arms furthers the twist and retains space for your heart and lungs. There will be some areas that are difficult to twist, while other areas are completely fluid. Mindfully walk from your tailbone to the crown of your head, observing how to create equanimity throughout your spine. Feel a broadness across your sacrum that soaks like watercolor all the way up your back. As you inhale, your entire body absorbs the color equally. As you exhale, the color saturation deepens, staining the very cells of your body.

ALTERNATE VIEW

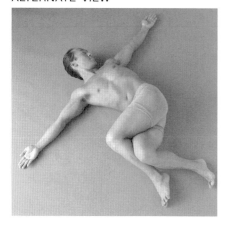

Observe the alignment of your spine—one continuous line from your tailbone to the crown of your head—at the same time respecting its natural curves. Feel as if your spine is a spiral staircase, evenly rising step by step and turning from the floor of your pelvis to the crown of your head.

If your right arm doesn't reach the ground, place your right hand on your lower back. The depth of the twist will continue its give and take with the rising and falling of your breath, your organs feeling as if they are sea sponges being squeezed and released by the opening and closing of your heart and lungs.

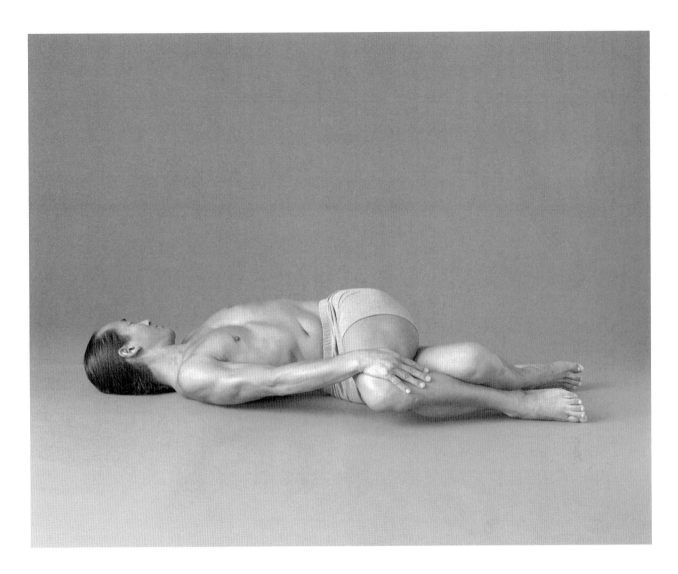

One Thing. Luxuriate in the supported unwinding of the binding of your spine. A cat in the warmth of the sun, moving innately.

Observation — the secret of dissolving the subtle tensions of the body and the mind.

Seated Crossed-Legged Twist

Parshva Sukhasana / 15 to 30 seconds

PREPARATION

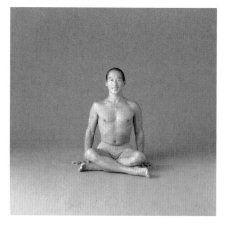

Start by sitting in a simple crossed-legged position with your right shin in front of your left shin. Bring your thighs toward each other so they are almost parallel, with your feet slightly to the outside of your thighs.

Next take both your hands behind you, lifting the front of your armpit-chest and lengthening your side waist. Ground your legs as your pelvis and spine feel an upward rising movement. The initiation of that extension comes from your pelvis sitting upright (your sitting bones wide and moving back, the top of your pelvis slightly forward).

DIRECTION OF MOVEMENT

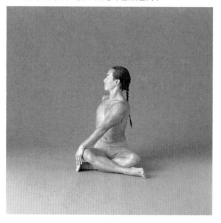

Now, take your left hand to your right knee and your right hand behind you, fingertips to the ground. From the extension of your spine, exhale and turn to your right. Start the twist from your pelvis, then let it spiral through your abdomen, your chest, and finally your head. Feel the foundation of your crossed legs as your pelvis rises into the full length of your spine, giving buoyancy and support to your heart and lungs. As your arms help you turn, stay broad in your collarbones and shoulder blades.

Feel a little give and a rise on your inhalation and a deeper twist on your exhalation. *Spun sugar. Cotton candy twisting around a paper cone.*

MODIFICATION

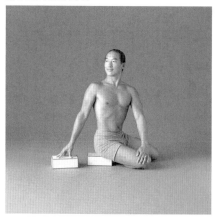

If your lower back is not in its natural curves when you sit with crossed legs, we recommend sitting on a block so that you can sit with ease. If your hand does not reach the ground easily as you turn, place another block under that hand. This modification allows your lower back to turn more freely, and it's healthier to turn from an elongated spine because your internal organs have more space and your diaphragm is not compressed, allowing you to breathe with ease. As your pelvis sits upright, your groins can release, allowing the foundation channel of your body to ground.

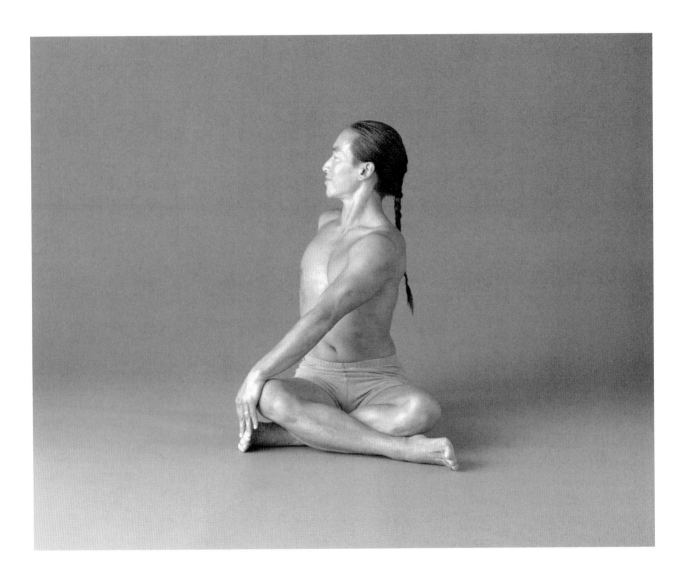

One Thing. Feel the broad strength of the foundation of your crossed legs connecting your twist to the gravitational pull of earth.

Support your heart, support your lungs, support your ability to sing.

Marichi's Pose 3

Marichyasana 3 / 15 to 30 seconds

DIRECTION OF MOVEMENT

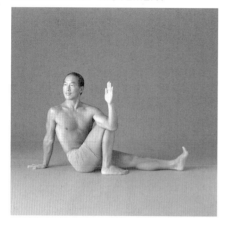

Start in Staff Pose (page 292), sitting with your legs extended forward vigorously and big toes touching. Bend your right leg into your chest, with your right heel in line with your right sitting bone. Then place your right hand behind you as you take your left upper arm to the outside of your right knee. Ground your legs to feed the upward motion of your spine.

Initiate the twist from the extension of your straight leg, allowing your left hip to move forward as your right groin deepens. Let your spine be carried upward like leaves in a swirling wind. As you come up against your resistance, use the leverage of your arms to begin to surrender the gripping around your spine and soften the determination of your mind and your neck.

ALTERNATE VIEW

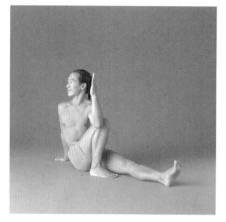

Funnel the grounding of your legs up through the channel of your spine. Your arms help both to move the dispersing energy upward and to elicit the movement of your shoulder blades firming into your back. *A regal neck. Eyes like a loving mother observing the play of your body.*

Feel the aliveness of your feet, for they are still the initiation of the grounding of your body. *Your spine emerging toward its natural curves.* Keep your front leg shinbone upright, as if it were the axis around which the energies of your body spin.

MODIFICATION

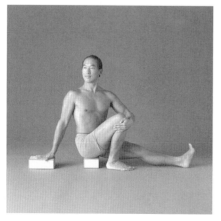

If you are tight in the hips, your spine may be thrown back from this positioning of your legs. This complicates the ease of your turn by forcing your back muscles to contract in an effort to keep your spine erect. Sitting on a block will allow you to decrease the amount of fold in your hips necessary to sit upright, so your torso muscles will be able to relax, easing the turn of your spine and freeing up your breath.

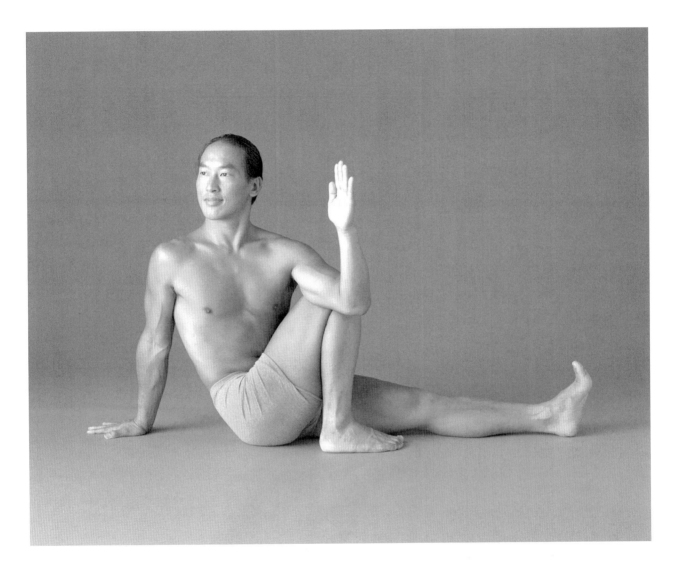

One Thing. Observe the resistance that arises from coming up against the limitations of your twist— don't smash yourself against the idea of the pose.

When you find a pose that's really difficult for you, be curious, be interested—let it unveil a deeper understanding about yourself.

Easy Lord of the Fishes Pose

Ardha Matsyendrasana 1 / 15 to 30 seconds

PREPARATION

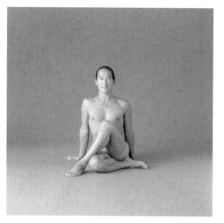

Bring your left leg into a simple crossed-legged position, with your left heel coming to the outside of your right hip. Then cross your right ankle over your left knee, placing the sole of your right foot on the ground, as shown in the photo. Take your left arm and hug your right leg, drawing your right knee toward your chest as you release your right hip toward the ground. Lean back on your right hand and extend your spine as you ground your legs. Inhale into the grounding of the pose and the length of your spine. Then exhale and begin to turn.

DIRECTION OF MOVEMENT

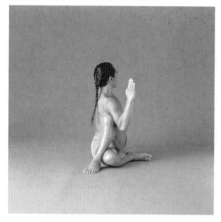

Release deeply in your right groin to feel the broad opening of your outer right hip. Allow your belly to recede and flow into the space between your spine and your right thigh. Drop your right hip downward, like water seeping into a crack, as your chest rises, like steam from the fires of your solar plexus.

The main opening in this twist is in your outer hips, augmented by the action of your arms. Don't force your head or neck. Exhale completely on each turn to fully surrender the tensions of your spine.

MODIFICATION

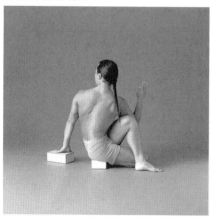

If you have tight hips and your pelvis and spine are thrown back from your legs as you take the leg position for this twist, we recommend sitting on a block so that you can focus on the twist and the opening of your hips. Place the block under both your sitting bones with your legs in the same position as shown for the preparation. Then move as closely as possible to the natural curves of your spine in this twist. This modification enables all of us to feel how the ease and length of the spine allow the twist to unfurl without congestion.

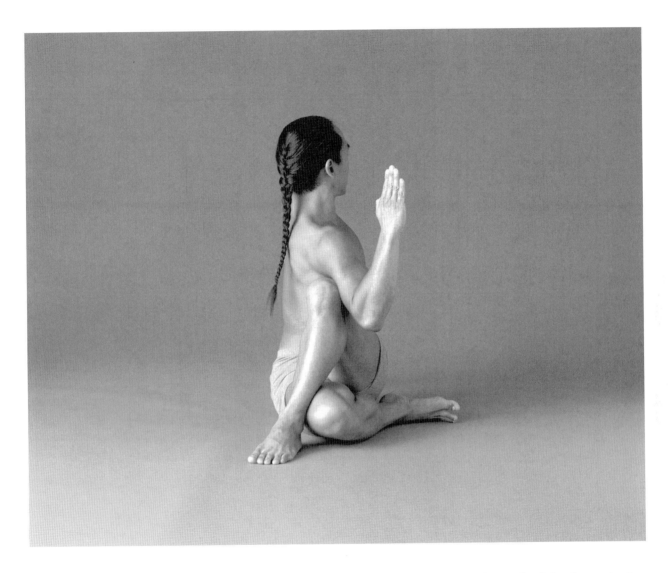

One Thing. Broad, open outer hips, watery, whirlpooling abdomen, flexing, flaring back body—spinning around yourself.

Your body is like a combination lock—when you find the numbers, it unlocks easily. And one of the numbers is moving toward the natural curves of your spine.

Back Bends

The poses in this section are good for energizing your entire being, opening your heart, and allowing vulnerability. At any time of the day when you need to rise out of lethargy, back bends will stir you up and stimulate your mind and body. They will also open your chest to bring ease to your breath and to bring you lightness and vitality.

strong legs
supple spine
open heart
broad mind

Use your arms and legs to open into the canopy of your chest. Let your heart and lungs remember innocence and receptivity. Your spine and your chest will work to regain their center from the habitual hunching you use to armor yourself from the world. Use the muscles of your back with fluidity and vigor to recenter yourself and drop all the unnecessary guarding.

You can do the poses in this section in the sequence in which they are presented as a short invigorating practice that will help awaken you and generate a creative surge in your body-mind.

Some questions to ask yourself while doing these poses:

- Am I jamming or locking any part of my spine?
- Can I sense the swooping arc of my body?
- Is there an ease to the pose, or am I straining?
- Am I remembering to breathe?

Cobra

Bhujangasana / 10 to 20 seconds

PREPARATION

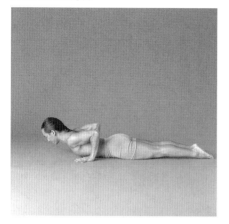

Start by lying on your belly. Draw your legs together, like the powerful tail of a reptile, as you lengthen your legs vigorously from your pelvis to the tips of your toes. Then place your hands by your middle ribs with your palms on the ground. Begin to elongate your waist and chest from the root of your legs, and press your hands down evenly as you draw your elbows close to the sides of your body.

Feel the length and suppleness of your spine emerging from the strength of your arms and legs.

DIRECTION OF MOVEMENT

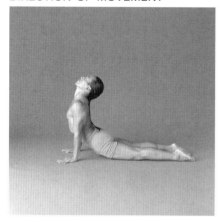

Pressing your hands into the ground, slowly weave your spine back and forth until it has reached its full, even arc. Straighten your arms only to the extent that they continue to support the length and opening of your spine without compression. Broaden your collarbones and lift your chest. Ground your legs as your pelvis and chest rise up and your head arcs back.

Use your arms mainly for lift and support while the muscles of your back and legs are responsible for the back bend. Feel the supple spine and sensual movements of a belly dancer.

MODIFICATION

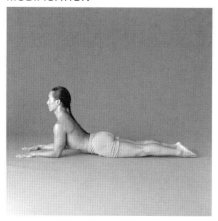

If your spine or the fronts of your hips are stiff, don't jam yourself into the full pose. Instead, prop yourself up on your elbows and spend some time allowing your spine to be languid from the lift of your chest sloping into the length of your legs. Let your arms support your chest as gravity pulls your legs down in the opposite direction. Because your arms don't have to be engaged, you can spend longer amounts of time searching for the ease of your spine as it bends backward.

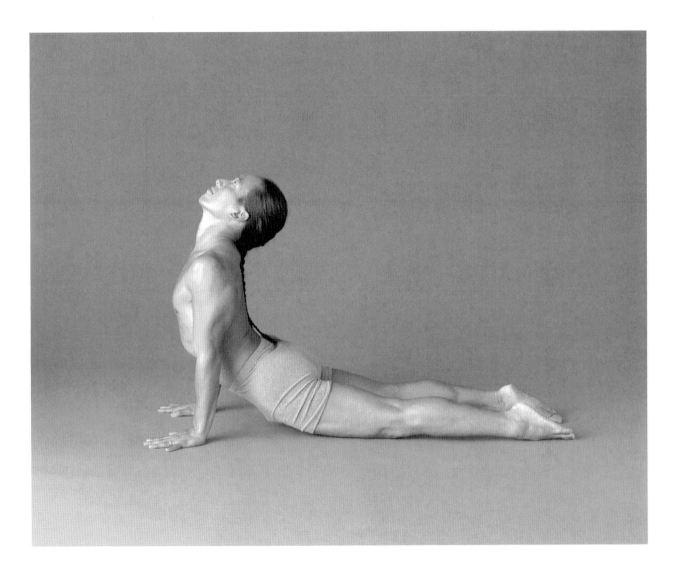

One Thing. Don't force. Be willing to spend time rediscovering the ease and articulation of your spine.

Move like a snake coming out of a basket—a subtle, sensuous, entrancing dance.

Push-up Pose

Chaturanga Dandasana (yes, we know this isn't a back bend, but it fits well into this sequence) / 3 to 5 seconds

PREPARATION (PLANK POSE)

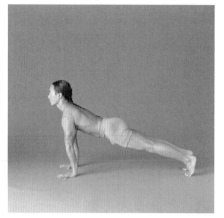

Start in Downward-Facing Dog (page 226). Then move into Plank Pose by bringing your shoulders forward until they are right over your hands, with your body in a straight line from your heels to your head. As you make the movement into Plank Pose, focus on maintaining the strength of your legs. Bring your pelvis in line between your legs and your torso as though you were in Mountain Pose. Gaze forward as the length of your front body moves into the openness of your chest, your back body stays broad but firm. Feel the vigor of your arms securely drawn into their sockets but pressing firmly into your hands. *The alignment of a staff with the agility of an animal.*

DIRECTION OF MOVEMENT

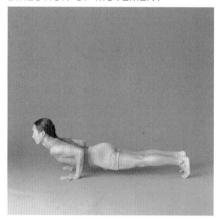

From Plank Pose, begin to bend your arms as far as you can (up to 90 degrees if possible) while maintaining the alignment of your body. Keep your elbows hugging close to your body while you lift your armpit-chest toward the direction of your head. *Hovering above the ground with the reptilian prowess of an alligator.*

Reach your sitting bones and tailbone toward your extending heels, like the alligator's long tail, while you lift your chest and forearms strongly from your rooted hands. Allow your upper chest to feel the natural urge to rise upward, like the surface of the sea beginning to surge into the powerful crest of a wave.

MODIFICATION

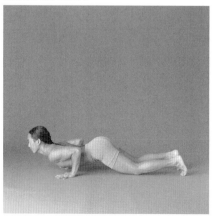

For those of you who have trouble bending your arms to 90 degrees while keeping your body in Plank Pose, we recommend that you bring your knees to the ground. This not only allows you to get a feeling for the position of your upper body in the full pose, but it is also a good intermediary step. Even though you bend your legs, retain their activity and integrity as the source of the pose. Keep your feet very active and your thighbones moving toward the back of your legs. Reach your sitting bones and tailbone toward your heels to elongate your lower back. Can you harness your arms into the core of your body without impinging on its openness? Periodically try extending your legs from this position.

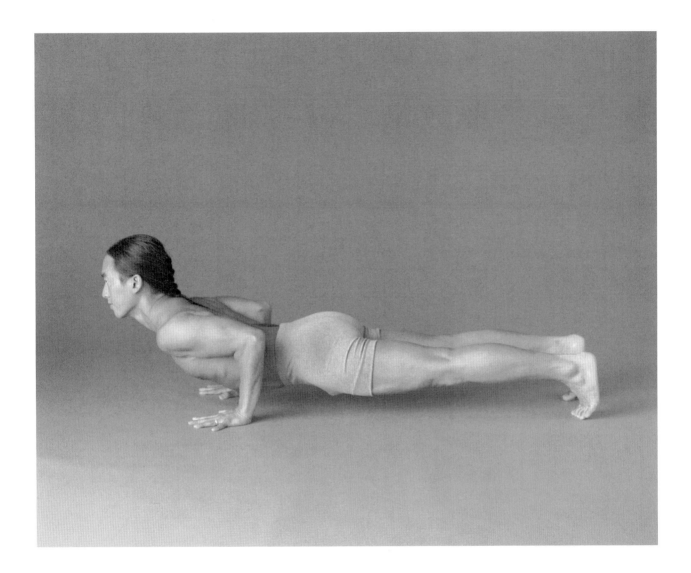

One Thing. Be willing to experience your weakness. Do the pose once now, and then do it again and again. Many of us are frustrated by the difficulty of Push-up Pose, but with repetition you can build up your strength very quickly. Yes, really.

Does your work need to come from determination?

Locust

Shalabhasana / 5 to 10 seconds

PREPARATION

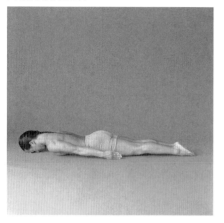

Start by lying on your belly with your legs together and extended and with your arms down by your side, reaching through your fingertips. Feel the relaxation that comes from having your belly on the ground, the extension that comes from lengthening your entire body from toe to head, and the absorption of your mind that comes from the depth of your breath.

Now bring your awareness to your soft underbelly between the intention of your legs and arms. How can you find full length without rigidity? How can you find breath without collapse?

DIRECTION OF MOVEMENT

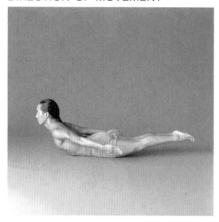

Without bending your legs, lift your legs up and back as you lift your chest forward and up. *Your entire body like the hull of a ship.* Then lift your arms parallel to the ground and look up with your head. Maintain the suppleness of your belly, and let your arms help lift your chest with their extension. At the same time sustain an expansive resonance to your chest.

Make sure the lift of your body is equaled by its length. The expansion of your chest is like the chest of a lion right before it roars. The lift of your head harmonizes with and augments the opening of your chest from the strength of your legs.

MODIFICATION

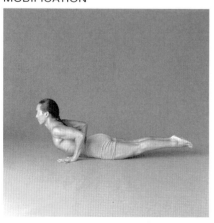

If this pose brings discomfort to your lower back, place your hands beside your chest, as in Push-up Pose. Press your hands into the ground, firming your shoulder blades into your back, with your arms right beside your body. Use your arms for extra support so that the muscles of your back can broaden from your spine. Also use your arms to move your chest forward, which will lengthen your spine as you back-bend. As you pull your chest forward, extend your legs vigorously in the opposite direction as you lift them. It's more important to create length than height in this pose. *Let your whole body hum.*

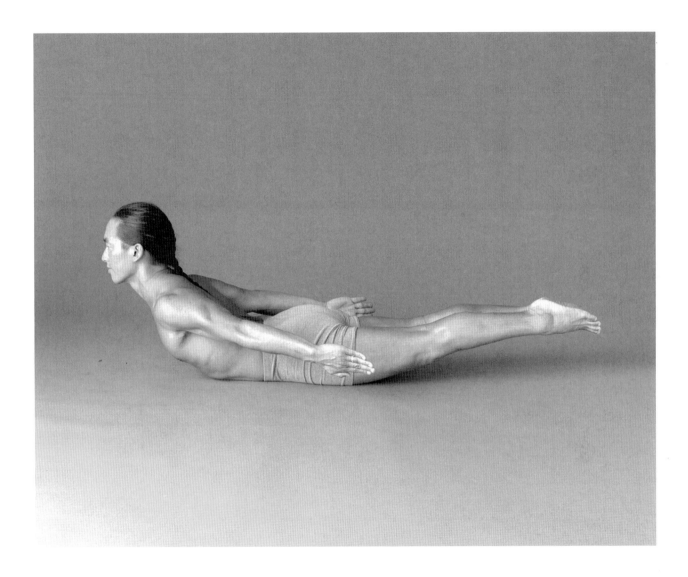

One Thing. Long, undulating spine—filled with breath—buoyant chest, and soaring legs.

Do it without a fever behind your eyes.

Bow Pose

Dhanurasana / 5 to 15 seconds

PREPARATION

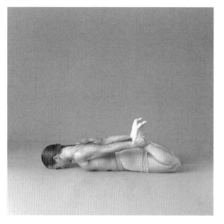

Start by lying on your belly. Bend your legs and hold on to your ankles, bringing your knees hips-distance apart. Try not to anticipate the pose; instead, follow the rise and fall of your breath. Relax your eyes and the back of your neck as you rest your forehead on the ground. Feel the relaxation at the front of your thighs as you allow the bottom of your pelvis to lift minutely from the ground. Elongate your waist and lower back. Let your tailbone feel as though it drops toward the ground as you open your upper chest.

DIRECTION OF MOVEMENT

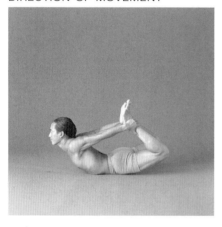

First lift your legs slowly; then lift your head and chest. As your legs, head, and chest lift, your arms will extend further as if they were the string of a bow. Lift your thighs strongly upward and into your hamstrings, and arc your chest forward and upward, letting your head and neck follow that graceful line. Broaden and open your back body as much as your front body. If your lower back pinches, don't lift as high, and try to get more length between the top of your buttocks and your back lower ribs. If your knees hurt, make sure you are not pushing the bottom of your pelvis into the ground, and play with the position of your feet (flexing or pointing them).

MODIFICATION

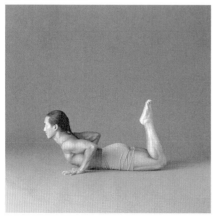

Some of you may not be able hold your ankles. In that case, place your hands beside your chest, as in Push-up Pose. Very slowly bend your legs, keeping your thighs parallel and dropping your tailbone toward the ground. With your arms pressing into the ground, move your chest forward and up. Follow with your head. Search your internal body to find an even, energetic arc that surges from your toes to the crown of your head. Feel your spine extend evenly, your heart open freely, and your legs work vibrantly. With soft eyes and a relaxed forehead, breathe easily.

Remember that it is the general shape and ease of the pose that is important, not straining at your physical edge.

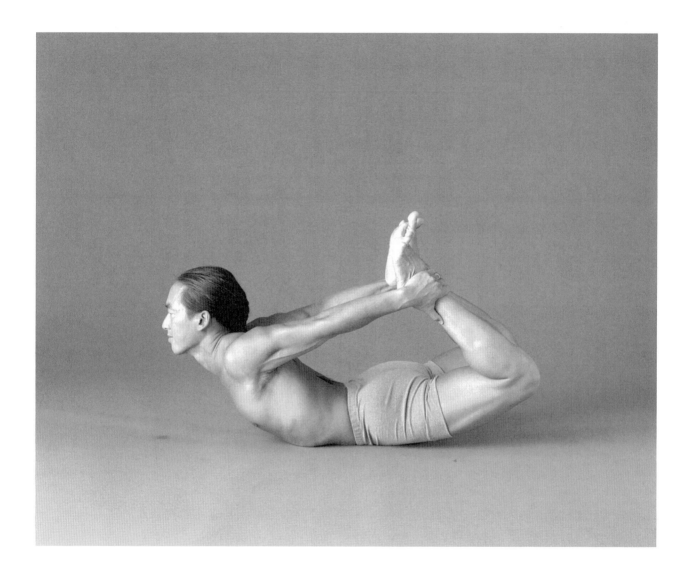

One Thing. Repetition and ease will allow you to deepen the pose far more profoundly than force and strain. So soften your determination and deepen your observation.

Let the difficulties course through your body—don't hold on to them.

Upward-Facing Dog

Urdhva Mukha Shvanasana / 5 to 15 seconds

PREPARATION

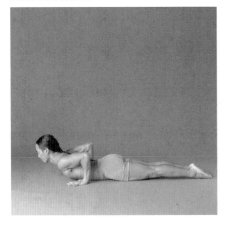

Start by lying on your belly with your legs together, the tops of your feet on the ground, and the soles of your feet pointing directly toward the ceiling. Extend your legs strongly and bring the heels of your hands alongside your middle ribs. Face your fingers in the direction of your head with your elbows close to your body. Next search for the length of your spine and the strength of your legs. Then, on an inhalation, press your hands into the ground, straighten your arms, and lift your chest into a back bend. Lift your legs from the ground and straighten them so that only the tops of your feet and your hands are touching the ground.

DIRECTION OF MOVEMENT

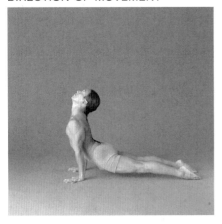

Press down strongly into the even placement of your hands as your arms draw into their sockets, and lift your chest vigorously. Keep the base of your neck soft and your legs strong. Create an even curve from the tips of your toes to the crown of your head, feeling every part of your spine contribute to that exhilarating arc. As your chest is lifted and opened, make sure that there is a quality of receptivity—a degree of suppleness and softness, a psychological vulnerability. *A lizard on a rock lifting its head to expose throat and belly to the sun.*

Let your breath resonate through your entire body. Exalt your heart and lungs.

MODIFICATION

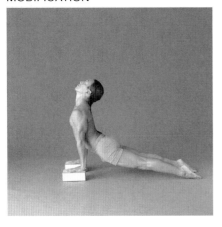

Upward-Facing Dog can be an extreme back bend, and some of you will get a pinching and discomfort in your lower back. If so, place your hands on blocks (one hand on each block), so your spine will not be required to bend as much. This will also make it easier on your wrists and enable you to lift your chest higher. Even though this pose should be done with great extension (that is, lift of your spine), there is the possibility of overextending. Therefore make sure there is a sense of relaxation in your back muscles, so they are supportive but not rigid. Allow yourself to play with the intensity of this pose, exploring the range between collapse and too much effort.

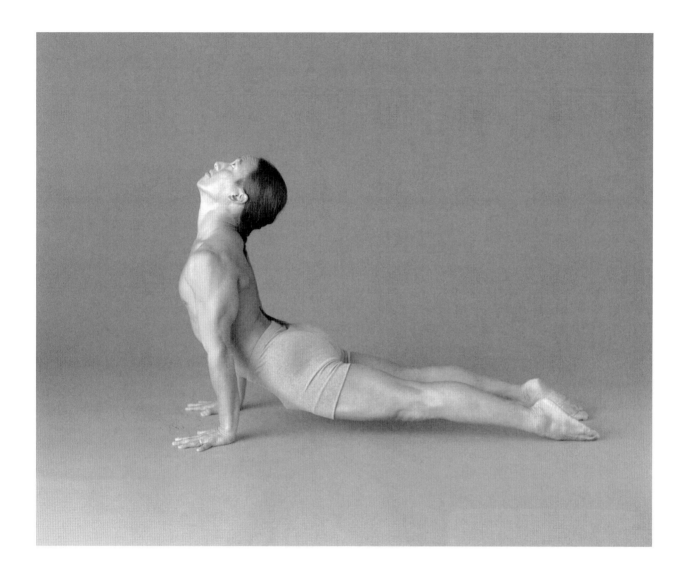

One Thing. A coyote opening the cavity of his chest, readying himself to let out a piercing, resonating howl.

Taking your time means listening to your inner body while you move your outer body.

Bridge Pose

Setu Bandha Sarvangasana / 10 to 20 seconds

PREPARATION

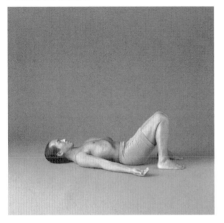

Start by lying on your back with your legs bent and the soles of your feet on the ground. Position your feet close to your hips, a little wider than hips-distance apart and with your toes turned in (pigeon-toed). Drop your knees toward each other as you ground your inner heels firmly downward. Keep your arms down by your sides. Relax your mind into your breath, and feel your inhalation move the broadness of your back body.

DIRECTION OF MOVEMENT

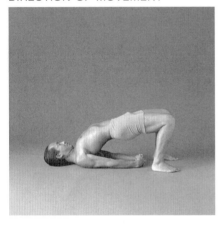

Press your feet and your arms downward and lift your pelvis, maintaining the broadness of your back body. Next interlace your fingers as you spin your arms under your chest. Then press your arms firmly into the ground as you lift your side chest with a soft, supple neck. Lift the outside of your hips from the strong press of your legs. Allow your thighbones to descend into the backs of your legs, and your belly to soften like that of a lazy cat on its back in the warm afternoon sun. Draw your inner legs toward your pelvis, and release your groins as your insteps and outer arches stay lifted. Feel the awakeness of your spine and the steadiness of your mind.

MODIFICATION

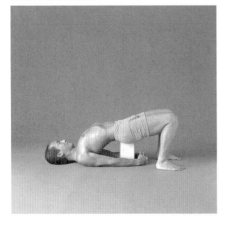

Place a block underneath your sacrum so that the weight of your pelvis is carried on it. This modification is useful for everyone because it enables you to sustain Bridge Pose for extended periods of time (two to five minutes). Sustaining Bridge Pose with a minimum of effort allows you to surrender more fully and enables your body to receive the benefits of a sustained pose (such as the calming of your nervous system and a quieting of your mind). By letting go of the restrictions, you can learn how to do this pose with far greater ease.

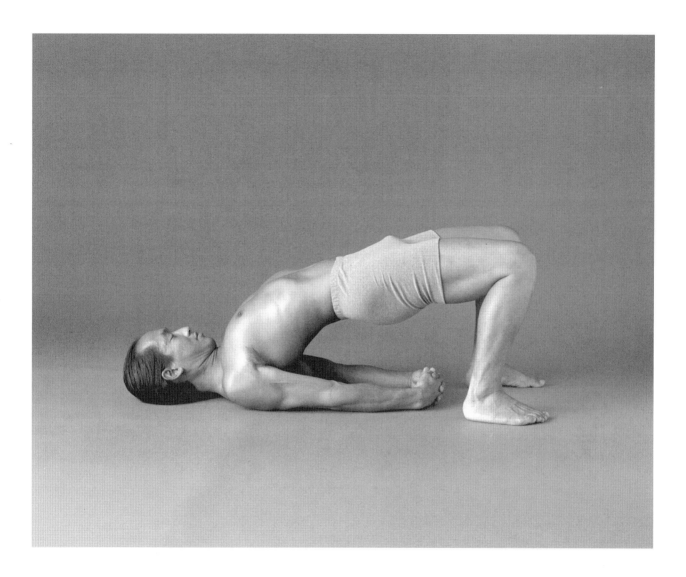

One Thing. Feel both the soothing and active qualities of this pose—soothing from the inversion of your body and active from the back-bending of your spine.

Drop the illusion that you are covering your heart—the secrets that you think you are hiding are exactly what show anyway.

—

Seated Poses

The poses in this section are good for opening your hips, bringing awareness to your habitual sitting posture, restoring your legs, and calming your mind. At the beginning of a practice, they give you space and time for your body and mind to center and drop into the activity at hand. At the end of a practice, they set you up for and flow smoothly into Relaxation Pose.

legs commanding attention
spine swaying subtly
arms floating gracefully
mind conversing with center

Come off your feet and use your legs as the pedestal of your body. Your contact with the ground increases a hundredfold, giving you that much more foundation from which to rise. Let your spine channel this energy through its suppleness, not its rigidity. Glide your arms from the height of your chest and the song of your heart. Balance your head over that breadth.

You can do the poses in this section in the sequence in which they are presented as a short meditative practice to bring yourself a moment of centering and quietness.

These are also good poses to integrate into your daily life. Hanging your legs down from a chair all the time swells them with stagnant blood and is actually uncomfortable. Try sitting on the floor as much as possible, and folding your legs into your chair at the movies, at dinner, and when talking to a friend. It's not easy to change your habits, but you will soon feel how your legs *want* to return to these natural positions. Bringing the sitting poses into your daily life will take out the stiffness in your hip joints, knees, and ankles. It will also help support and strengthen your spine.

Some questions to ask yourself while doing these poses:

- How do my knees feel?
- Can I maintain the natural curves of my spine?
- Am I rigid or fluid?
- Do I feel my breath rising and falling with ease?

Simple Crossed Legs

Sukhasana / 30 seconds to 2 minutes

PREPARATION

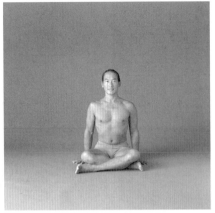

Sit with your legs crossed, taking note of which shin you naturally place in front of the other (alternate regularly). Now move your feet underneath your knees so that your shinbones are parallel to each other. Bring your knees close enough together so that your legs form a square. Use your hands to pull your buttocks flesh and your sitting bones wide and away from your knees. Place your hands or fingertips down beside you on the floor. Now press firmly into the ground to help elongate your waist, and feel the lift of your chest and the curves of your spine. Make sure this effort does not create rigidity but allows the movement of your breath to be received with ease.

DIRECTION OF MOVEMENT

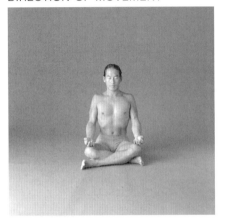

Place your hands on your thighs with your palms facing up. Then draw your arms up into their sockets as your shoulder blades release down your back. Feel the broadness of your back muscles fanning from the center of your spine and the lift of your front body from your groins to your collarbones. Float your head above your heart, and realize that balance and centering are a constant dialogue. *Head over chest, chest over pelvis, pelvis over legs, legs over earth.* What physical effort can you let go of without collapsing? Continue to follow your breath—where is it moving and how? Now scan your body from feet to head, and notice the areas that are vague or difficult to feel compared with the areas that are full of sensation.

MODIFICATION

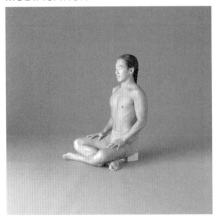

For many of us, because of the tightness of our legs and hips, it is impossible to sit flat on the ground and maintain the natural curves of our spine. Therefore we recommend you sit on a block or folded blanket that is high enough to allow your pelvis to be upright. Use your hand to check whether there's a slight sway in your lower back. If your knees are high off the ground, place folded blankets underneath them. You can also sit with your back against a wall, so your back muscles can relax. The wall also reminds you to align your torso so the back of your head, your shoulder blades, the middle of your sacrum, and your sitting bones are in contact with the wall.

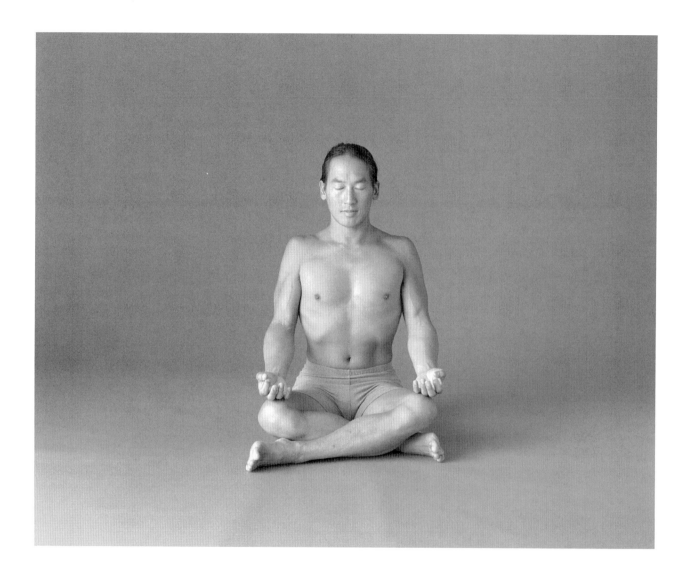

One Thing. The solitude of sitting allows you to touch the expanse of the universe.

What we're doing here is honing the mind so we can peer more deeply into existence.

Hero Pose

Virasana / 30 seconds to 2 minutes

DIRECTION OF MOVEMENT

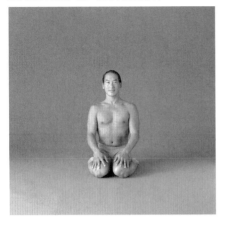

Bring your knees close together, with your feet a little wider than hips-distance apart and the soles of your feet facing the ceiling and extending straight back from your shins. Next begin to move back toward a sitting position, and as you do so, use your hands to pull your calf muscles down toward your heels and slightly out toward the sides. Allow the tops of your thighbones to descend toward the ground as your spine finds its natural curves and your side waist lengthens into the lift of the sides of your chest. *The coiled spring of your legs unleashing into the light of your spine.*

ALTERNATE VIEW

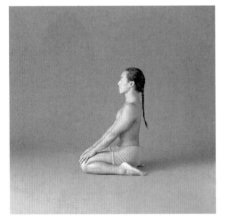

For most of us, our sitting bones won't touch the ground without creating strain in our knees. Therefore it is essential to sit on a block or folded blanket in this pose unless you can sit firmly and with ease on the ground without the prop. Move your inner thighs toward your groins, and draw the arches of your feet toward the backs of your knees. If your knees still feel uncomfortable, use your hands to lift each knee slightly and pull the skin of your kneecaps away from your shins and toward the tops of your thighs.

For most of us, this pose now seems unnatural and irritating, but as a child this was probably your most common sitting position for playing games on the floor (remember cards, marbles, and jacks?).

MODIFICATION

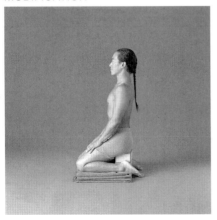

If your main tightness is not in the fronts of your thighs but in the fronts of your ankles and feet, you will feel an excessive pull at both your ankles and knees. You can modify the pose by placing a stack of folded blankets under your shins and dangling your feet off the edge. This modification, along with the block under your hips, makes it possible for you to sit for longer periods of time because it gives your legs and hips time to evolve slowly into a deeper fold. Over time, as your legs become more supple, you can reduce the height of your support. It is important to attend to your restrictions yet at the same time be curious about exploring them.

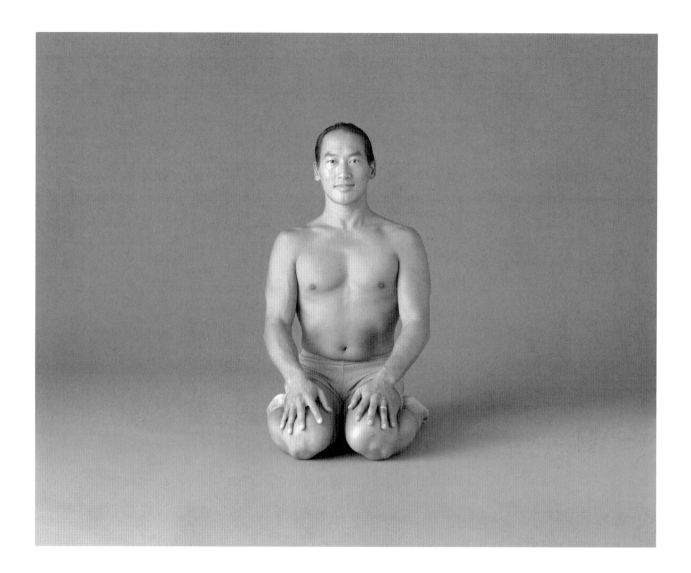

One Thing. Great relief for the muscles of your legs, which hold so much tension and activity (Nepalese Sherpas, whose legs are among the strongest in the world, are often seen resting in this pose).

Create a sense of receptivity before you start to practice. Then there's a possibility for observation.

Lion Pose

Simhasana / 3 to 5 roars

DIRECTION OF MOVEMENT

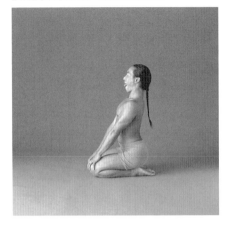

Start by sitting on your heels with your hands on your knees. Feel a great lift in your chest, as if you were a lion about to roar. And let that lift of your chest come from the full arch of your spine, from your tailbone to your chest, with the side walls of your chest thrusting forward and upward between your arms. With your hands holding your knees, gaze at the tip of your nose, letting your eyes cross, and stick your tongue out, reaching for your chin. Open your jaw wide, feeling the full stretch of your face. Now roar three times, as loudly as you want, inhaling through your nose and roaring through your mouth. Allow the vibrations of your inner body coming from the depths of your intestines to reverberate throughout the room.

What's there to say?

ALTERNATE VIEW

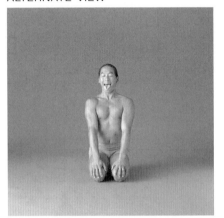

MODIFICATION

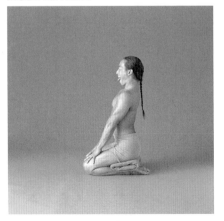

If you cannot sit comfortably on your heels, place a rolled-up or folded blanket between your heels and buttocks. Put your hands on your thighs (they won't reach your knees when you sit raised up like this). Then press them into your thighs as you extend your claws. Extend your waist and lift your chest from the press of your hands as you feel the arch of your spine unfurl from its sleeping coil. Gaze at the tip of your noise, letting your eyes cross. Open your jaw wide as you reach for your chin with the tip of your tongue. From the ferocity of your legs rising into the channel of your spine, unleash three roars from your belly through your chest and out the cavity of your mouth.

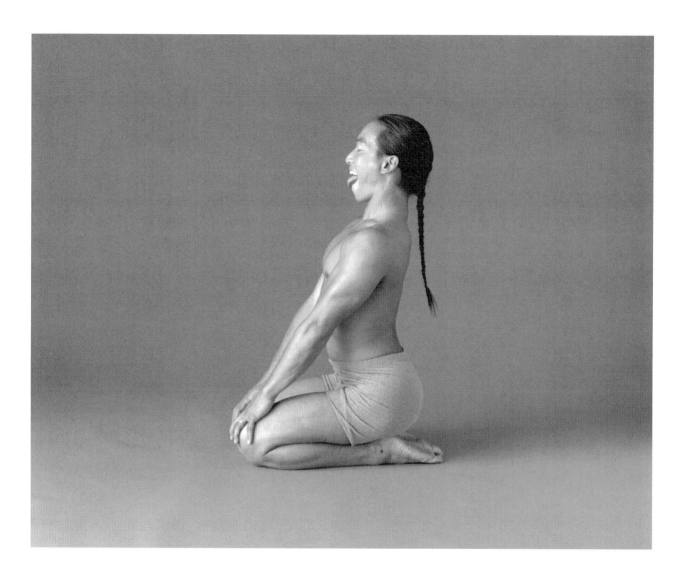

One Thing. Feel the intensity of your body, and transform that into sound.

Allow yourself to be empty—then your voice will emerge.

Cobbler's Pose

Baddha Konasana / 30 seconds to 2 minutes

DIRECTION OF MOVEMENT

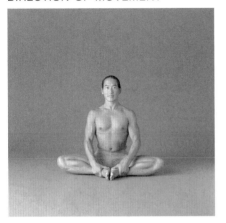

Start by sitting with the soles of your feet together. Now hold your ankles and draw your feet toward or to your hips, letting your legs drop open. Lightly press your heels together, as if you were holding something between your feet, and feel your inner knees moving away from each other. Deepen your sacrum forward as you use your arms to help lift your chest. Elongate your torso as the muscles right around your spine broaden and relax. Drop the tops of your thighs out of your pelvis and down toward the ground, feeling your pelvis float upward from the broad grounding of your legs. As your arms pull, feel an ease at the back of your neck, your head like a buoy on the currents of your breath.

MODIFICATION 1

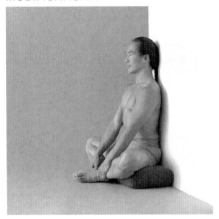

If you are thrown back by tightness in your hips and are unable to right your pelvis, try sitting on a block against the wall. This modification allows your spine and your pelvis to sit upright with ease, enabling you to focus on releasing your legs. You will then be able to hold this pose for longer periods of time without strain or stress. Start by sitting on the block. Then move your sitting bones as close to the wall as possible, feeling your lower back move away from the wall. The middle of your sacrum, the middle of your back, and the back of your skull should be the dominant points of contact with the wall. Use the wall not only to support your body weight but to remind you to lengthen and widen your back body. *Let go and rise up.*

MODIFICATION 2

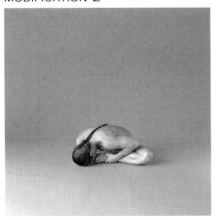

As you draw yourself forward, press the baby toe side of your heels together. If the insides of your feet come apart naturally, that's okay, but support the outsides of your ankles with your fingers to keep them more aligned. As you pull with your arms, deepen your groins and feel a gentle arc throughout your spine. Even though you are in a forward bend and even though you are pulling with your arms, keep your chest broad and extending forward. Allow your efforts in the pose to go toward releasing more deeply in your hip sockets. It's more important to maintain the extension in your spine than to try to bring your head to the ground. *With an ease of breath and a completion of surrender . . .*

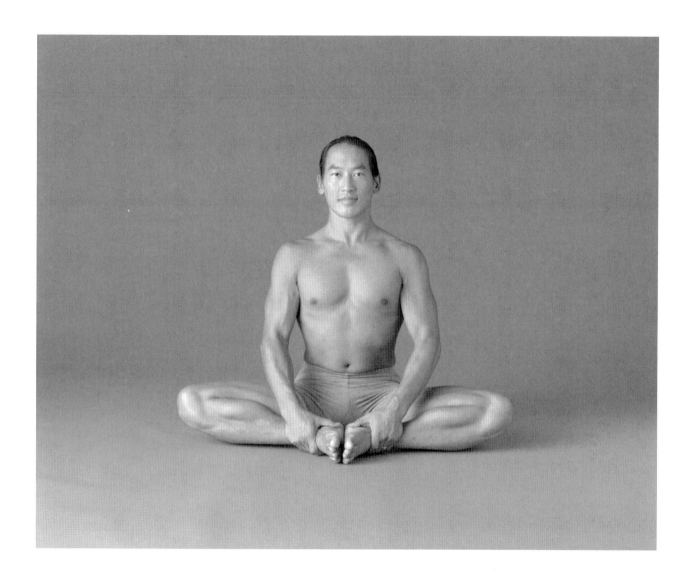

One Thing. Where exactly is the resistance in your pelvis that is not allowing your legs to fall open and your spine to soar upward?

If you can't seem to understand something — walk around it, play with it, sit with it.

Staff Pose

Dandasana / 10 to 20 seconds

DIRECTION OF MOVEMENT

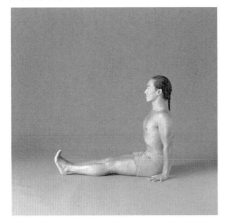

Bring your legs together, feeling your alive, tactile feet and vibrant toes. Press the back of your thighs, the back of your calves, and your heels strongly and evenly down into the ground. And yet even as you press strongly into the ground, make sure that you don't dampen the vibrancy of your legs. Press your hands into the ground and lift your chest. You can gauge the amount of effort you put into the grounding of your legs and the lifting of your chest by observing the depth of the absorption of your breath.

From the action of your legs and arms, lengthen your waist. Imagine your legs are buried in the sand and you are lifting your torso to break free. *Earth of legs, sky of chest.*

MODIFICATION 1

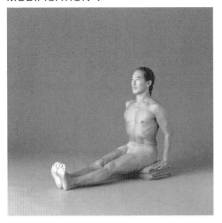

This modification is for people who have tight hamstrings and therefore have a difficult time maintaining a vertical pelvis with straight legs. Sitting on a block allows you to extend your spine while you ground your legs. Otherwise your spine feels chained to the earth. The prop helps you find some liberation for your lower back and pelvis, and understand that the roots are your legs and the beginning of the tree trunk is the base of your pelvis.

Extend your side waist into the broadening of your chest, with your collarbones moving from the sternum out to the shoulders. Your sternum should be lifted but relaxed.

MODIFICATION 2

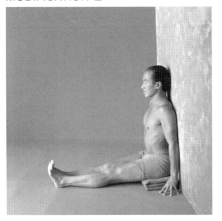

This modification is for people who have back problems and need extra support for their spines. The wall provides support so your back muscles don't have to overwork and allows you to sustain the pose for longer periods of time, so you can explore the more subtle energies moving in this pose. With your back on the wall, feel your back muscles broadening from your spine. Feel the juxtaposition between your legs pressing against the ground and your back body lengthening up the wall. *Broad, strong legs converging into the shimmering of the spine.*

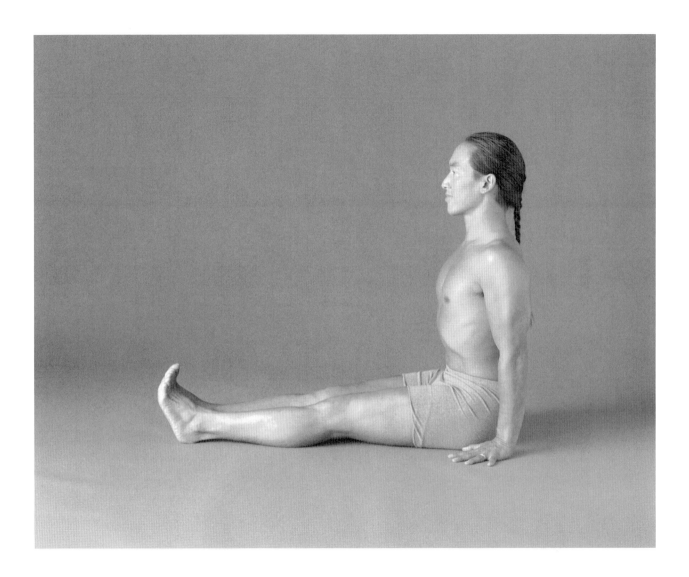

One Thing. A centaur. Your legs with the strength of a horse and your human torso rising effortlessly from that animal grace.

The physical is not mundane—it's just as much of a mystery as the soul.

Forward Bends

The poses in this section are good for soothing your nervous system, opening up your back body, rejuvenating your sense organs, and turning your mind inward. Forward bends are perfect poses for resting a weary body and settling an overactive mind, especially before going to bed.

legs opening completely
back body resting deeply
exhalation lengthening smoothly
mind receding softly

Be patient in letting yourself unwind. Feel your exhalation seep completely out of your body. Let your mind begin to cool down like the beginning of a spring evening. Sense a feeling of security as your body folds into itself. Let the poses be like reflections in a still pool.

You can do the poses in this section in the sequence in which they are presented as a short unwinding practice to let the worries and traumas of the day fall away.

Some questions to ask yourself while doing these poses:

- Am I bending forward mainly from my hips and letting my spine follow without force?
- Is my spine equal in its arc?
- Do my heart and lungs still have space and support?
- Am I staying sensitive to the slow release of the tightness in my legs?

Child's Pose

Balasana / 15 seconds to 2 minutes

PREPARATION

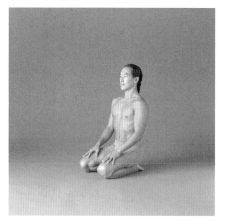

Start by sitting on your heels with your big toes together and your knees slightly apart. Press your hands down on the tops of your thighs, and feel the downward movement of your thigh-bones against your calves and the stretching of your shins into the extension of your feet. Now elongate your spine from the grounding of your legs and see how completely you can drop your sitting bones onto your heels. You might be surprised how much your legs fold, with time and a little persistence. Your leg muscles can be both strong and supple.

DIRECTION OF MOVEMENT

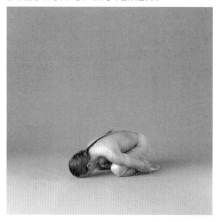

Maintaining the fold of your legs, release your spine over your legs, placing your forehead on the ground and your arms by your legs. Feel most of the weight of your torso drape over your legs as your neck and head rest easily, your body like an accordion that with gravity is slowly folding into its complete compactness. Adjust the distance between your knees so your weight falls back toward your heels and not on your neck and head. Child's Pose is one of the most amazing forward bends, immediately comforting your mind and body as it turns you inward. You can feel completely nurtured in the silence of being, an embryo deep in the belly of your mother.

MODIFICATION

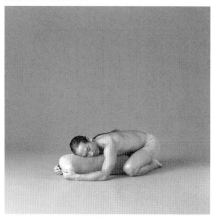

If your legs do not fold deeply enough for your hips to touch your heels, lay your torso over a bolster. Position the bolster between your legs so it supports your torso but does not separate your feet. Rest your belly, head, and chest evenly. This modification lifts your head to at least the height of your hips. For comfort in your neck and face, you may need to turn your head to one side.

This modification can often create a deeper restoration because your front body is in tactile contact—feeling full support from the bolster. *A baby sleeping, its body nestling against the breasts of its mother.*

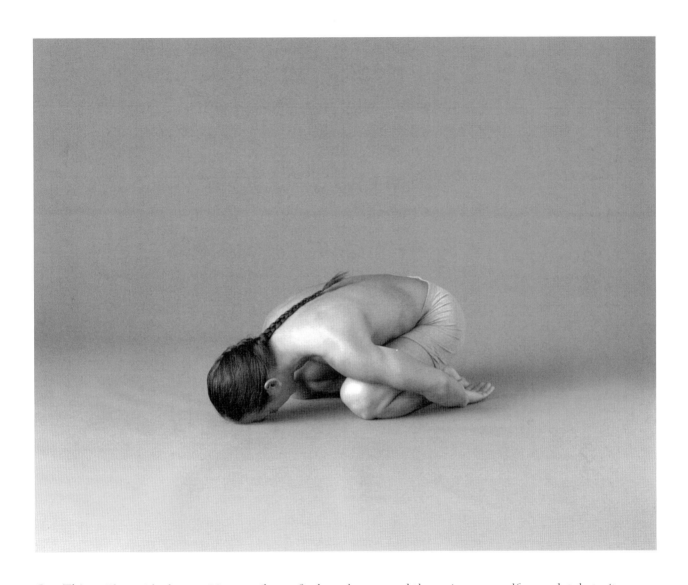

One Thing. Play with the position until you find total ease, and then give yourself completely to it.

Fall in love with subtlety.

Crossed-Legged Forward Bend

15 to 30 seconds

PREPARATION

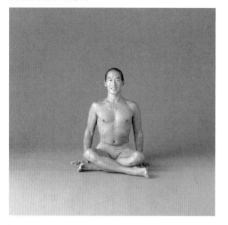

Start by sitting with your right ankle and calf in front of your left (in other words, don't stack your ankles) and with your thighs almost parallel. Place your hands beside your hips, and extend your waist from your sitting bones up through your chest.

Ground your legs downward, and rotate them so your knees turn away from each other. Feel as much broadness to your back body as length to your front body, being careful not to extend so much that you stifle your breath.

DIRECTION OF MOVEMENT

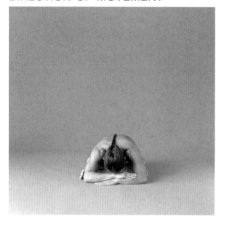

Release forward on an exhalation, placing your arms on the ground and your forehead on your arms. As your legs continue to ground downward and to rotate externally, let your spine gracefully undulate into a passive rest, releasing any habitual tension. Be especially observant of the surrender of your neck muscles to feel the true weight of your head being carried by your arms. Make any small movements that enhance the ease of your breath, the broadness of your neck, and the quietness of your mind. Feel your back body spread from your spine like a heavy quilt thrown over you for warmth and security. And turn into yourself as a child often does when he curls up for sleep.

MODIFICATION

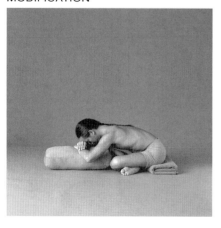

If your head and forearms don't reach the ground easily in this forward bend, sit on a blanket or a block to elevate your pelvis and place a bolster or a chair under your head and arms. This modification will allow your spine to stay more extended. There will also be less congestion in your abdomen, which will free up your breathing and allow the forward bend to be more restorative. The blanket under your hips will also help propel you forward, so be more attentive to grounding your legs downward not by pushing your knees down but by pressing your upper thighs down. *Your mind nestled in the silence of your inner body.*

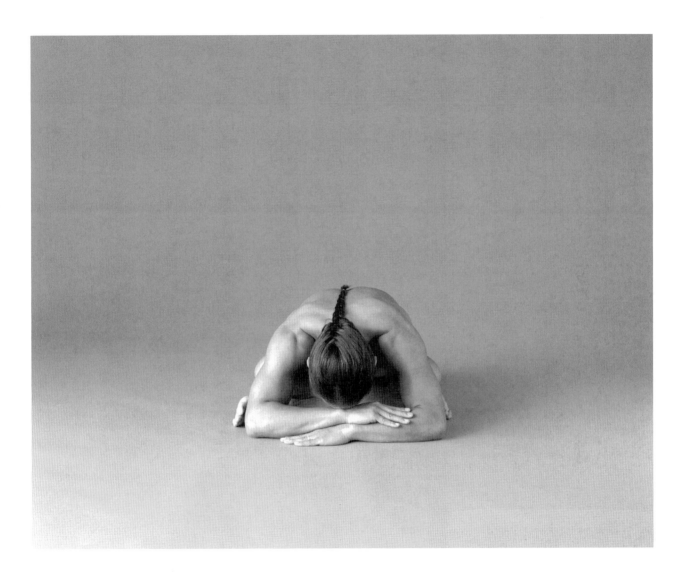

One Thing. Forward folding coupled with a crossed-legged position opens up two of the most support-ive areas of your body: your back and your hips. Feel them release as your mind and body are carried by the support of the earth.

A flower doesn't unfold with difficulty—it's in its nature.

One-Legged Forward Bend

Janushirshasana / 15 to 30 seconds

PREPARATION

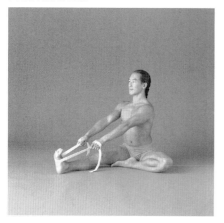

Start in Staff Pose (page 292). Now fold your left leg into your torso, bringing your left heel as close to your left sitting bone as possible. Then drop your left leg open to the side.

Place a strap around the arch of your right foot. Lift your chest from your strongly descending legs. Lengthen your side waist, feeling that length coming more from the strength of your arms and legs than from the muscles of your back. Feel your sitting bones spread back and wide, away from the heel of your straight leg. Deepen the fold of your bent leg by moving the top of your pelvis forward toward the heel of your bent leg.

DIRECTION OF MOVEMENT

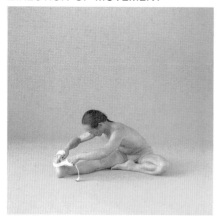

Spill your pelvis forward over your straight leg, followed by your lower back, your middle back, your upper back, and finally your head. If you can reach your foot easily, let go of the strap and draw your spine forward with the bending of your arms. Ground down through your legs as you propel your chest forward from your belly. Sense the vitality of the energy you draw from your legs into the reach of your spine. As you feel the resistance of the back of your legs—your hamstrings and your calves—dissolve their tension and breathe into the physical sensations that are arising. Instead of fighting with the backs of your legs, sit with their nature.

MODIFICATION

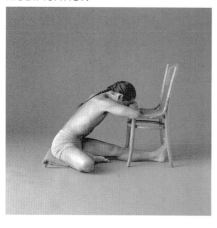

If you find this forward bend coming primarily from your lower back instead of evenly from the back of your legs, your hips, and your entire back body, sit on a blanket or block and place your head on a chair. This modification helps create equanimity in the pose—the chair takes the weight of your head and neck from your lower back, and the blanket elevates your pelvis, allowing it to spill forward more easily. For anyone, these modifications make the pose more restorative, enabling you to focus on the more subtle sensations and directions of movement in the posture. Be aware of how your breath is being absorbed into your back body.

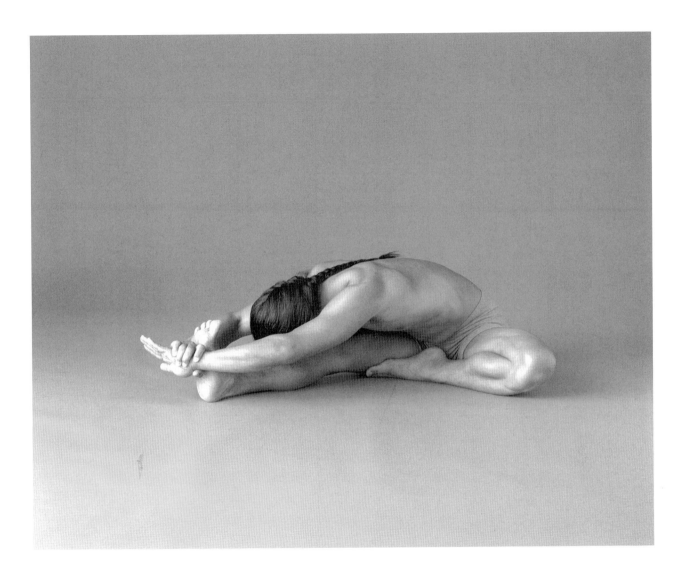

One Thing. As your resistance arises from your physical limitations and your mental desires, meet them both with observation and passion by extending strongly over your straight leg as your breath and mind stay at ease.

Relax and pay attention—don't harden and pay attention.

Marichi's Pose 1

Marichyasana 1 / 15 to 30 seconds

PREPARATION

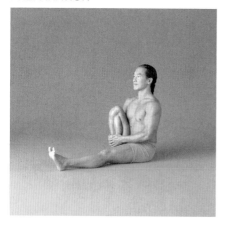

Start in Staff Pose (page 292), with your legs together, your toes flexed and wide, your heels reaching, and the arches of your feet drawing from those foundations up the stem of your legs into the length of your spine. Press your legs downward, feeling the energetic vibrations circulating from feet to hips and hips to feet. Take the vibrations of your legs and channel them up through your spine as you use your arms to enhance the lift and broadness of your chest up to your neck and head. Draw your right knee into your chest, using your hands at your ankle to pull your right heel as close as possible to your right sitting bone.

DIRECTION OF MOVEMENT

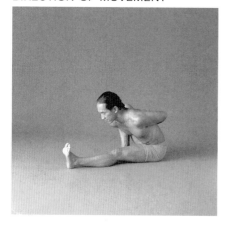

Hug your right leg, and, from the strength of your legs, propel your body upward. This shape will naturally broaden the back of your torso. From this broadness, feel the extension of your front body from the bottom of your pelvis to your collarbones. As you pull with your arms, gather the energy of your legs into the emergence of your chest and the regal carriage of your neck and head. Make sure that you don't pull your shoulder girdle downward on your heart and lungs. Instead, feel your arms give buoyancy to the palace of your heart and suppleness to the base of your neck. Keep accentuating the uprightness of your pelvis as it folds deeply against the right thigh.

MODIFICATION

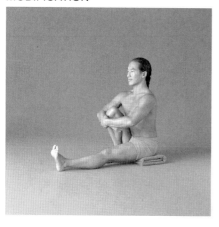

If your hips are tight and your pelvis is thrown back from your bent leg, sit on a blanket or block, so your back muscles will not have to tighten to move your spine upright. The blanket will also allow the foot of your bent leg to press more strongly into the ground. As you sit on the blanket, make sure you do not jam the knee of your straight leg toward the ground, but instead draw your muscles up along the bone from your foot to your hip. Through this modification, you begin to understand and change the relationship between your lower back, sacrum, and hip sockets. As you sit on the blanket, your lower back and sacrum take a more natural position, demanding that your hip sockets come to their natural flexibility.

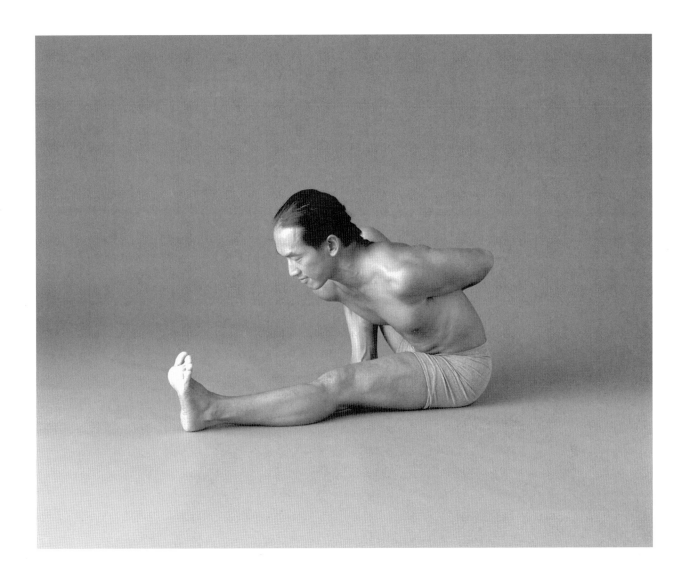

One Thing. The hip joint is the dividing line between the energy of your legs rooting downward and your spine flying upward.

Let your arms and legs be the tributaries of the river of your spine.

Seated Forward Bend

Paschimottanasana / 15 to 45 seconds

DIRECTION OF MOVEMENT

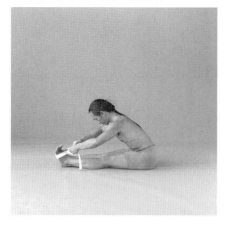

Start in Staff Pose (page 292), holding onto your feet with your hands or a strap. Then, with strong legs, extend your side waist and slowly release forward. Release your groins as your sacrum moves deeper toward the front of your body. Keep your sitting bones wide as your tailbone relaxes between them, and let your legs be two strong energy channels. Round your spine evenly like the curve of a tortoise shell. Continue to move your chest forward by pulling with your arms—elbows lifted out to the sides—so that your heart and lungs are supported and open. Your head is subjugated through the equal opening of your back body and the turning inward of your senses toward your core. *Deep reprieve in the midst of a great battle.*

MODIFICATION 1

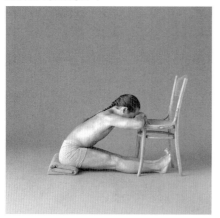

Place your head and arms on the seat of the chair, and feel its coolness on your forehead as you release the knots of effort rising from your legs and spine. Rest your weary soul over the strength and vitality of your legs as your breath finds the completion of the exhalation. Let the chair help you realize that the essential aspect of the forward bend is not how close your head comes to your legs but how completely you abandon yourself in rest. For those of you who tend to be aggressive in forward bends, this modification will teach you to surrender more than to struggle.

MODIFICATION 2

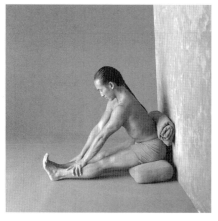

If you have tight hamstrings that prevent you from being able to release forward with ease, you can sit on a bolster or block with your back against a wall. Start by sitting on a bolster in Staff Pose, and bring your back as close to the wall as possible. Next place a rolled blanket between your lower back and the wall. The blanket roll wedged between your back and the wall will set up the proper release to allow your body to move more deeply into the forward bend without straining your back. By elevating your pelvis, the bolster allows you to use gravity to spill your pelvis over your legs. The wall and the blanket further that release by reminding you to widen the muscles of your back away from your spine.

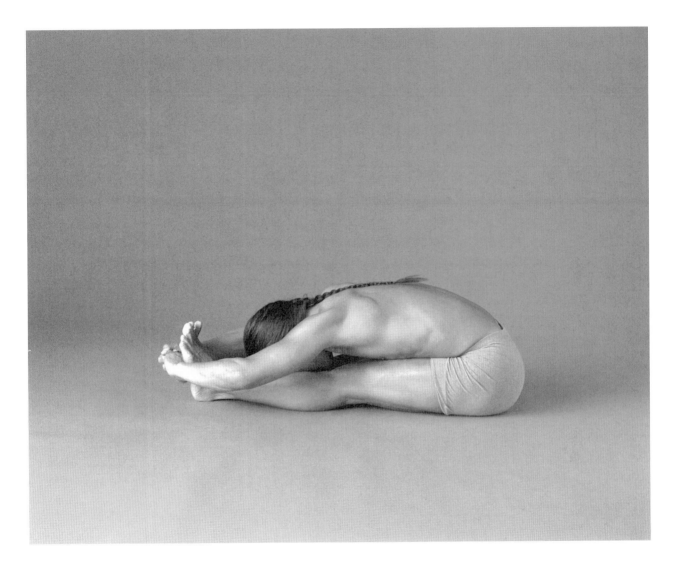

One Thing. Bending forward with both legs straight brings up a strong physical resistance—emotional frustration, physical discomfort, and mental agitation. Meet these difficulties with breath and presence of mind.

Wait for a forward bend as if you are river rafting and charting your course before you run the water. Look at your legs, and navigate before you dive.

Wide-Angle Forward Bend

Upavishta Konasana / 15 to 45 seconds

PREPARATION

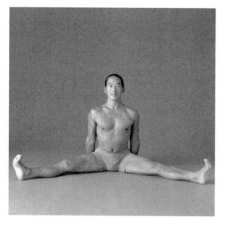

Start by sitting with your legs open wide—your knees and toes pointing directly upward. Then take your hands behind you, your fingertips touching the ground. Streamline your leg muscles along the bone, drawing up from your arches to your pelvis. As you feel the full length of your leg bones reaching from sitting bones to heels, widen your toes like opening a fan. Press your legs downward so your calf muscles and hamstrings begin to soften and spread like liquid soaking onto the ground. From the touch of your fingertips behind you, undulate your spine with your breath into its full, unadulterated length.

DIRECTION OF MOVEMENT

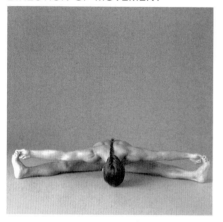

Continue to bring your attention to your grounded legs as you slowly bend your body forward like bamboo in a heavy wind, staying intensely rooted to the earth while your head and body soften. Feel both the vulnerability from the spread and stretch of your inner legs and the security arising from the protection provided to your vital organs by your back. Relish this unusual combination—the turning inward of the forward bend along with the wide spreading of your body on the ground elicits a deep surrender, like looking over a vast desert landscape in the light of early morning.

MODIFICATION

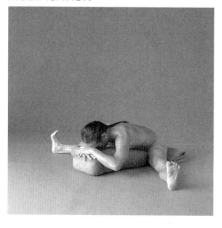

If you are tight in the hamstrings and the insides of your legs or have lower back problems, you can do this pose by sitting on the edge of a folded blanket. Extending your spine, come forward onto a bolster or a chair, whichever allows for ease in your lower back.

Maintain strong activity in your legs to keep your knees fully extended and the backs of your thighs pressing toward the ground—this helps you realize the full length of your spine. Observe the surrender of your body and the movement of your breath. Move your breath into your back body as your front body stays supported and open. *Fall into the depth of yourself.*

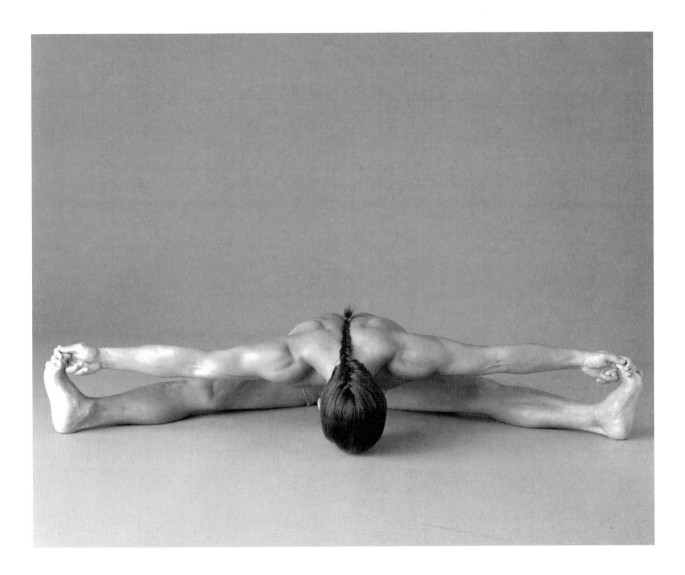

One Thing. Keep pinpointing the areas of physical and emotional resistance, knowing that with time and practice you can turn this frustrating pose into one that is enjoyable and soothing.

Feel your breath falling onto your back body as if it were being pelted by rain.

Restorative Poses

The poses in this section are good for giving yourself much-needed rest. They are great transition poses, taking you from a day of work to an evening at home or from a busy week into an open, unplanned weekend. Sometimes you need them as much at the beginning of your practice as at the end. For example, you might want to start a practice with Legs Up the Wall Pose to help you begin with quiet observation before moving into more vigorous poses. And always end your practice with one of the restorative poses to allow for integration and digestion of all that you've felt and learned.

> *body supported completely*
> *breath rising and falling easily*
> *mind wandering freely*

As you let the boundaries of your body and your mind dissipate, feel the free falling of your entire being as you drop your bones to the earth. Your exhalations feel like long sighs as you give up for the moment your aspirations, your identifications, your tribulations, and your longings.

You can do the poses in this section in the sequence in which they are presented as a practice that will allow you to let go, let down, and just be. Let your breath dominate your existence as you feel what you consider the solid world melt into the ever-changing, amorphous universe.

A question to ask yourself while doing these poses:

- Is there an end to letting go?

Restorative Twist

30 seconds to 2 minutes

PREPARATION

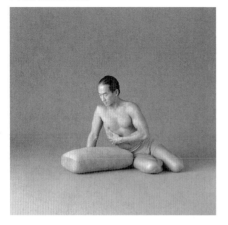

Start by sitting on your heels. Place a bolster to your right, with the short end closest to your hip. Next slide your hips to the right so your right hip comes to the ground, as you lean onto the bolster. Position your legs so that your left lower shin is in the instep of your right foot. Turn to face the bolster and pull it against your hip. Elongate your right waist by moving your right ribs toward the far end of the bolster. From here, turn your chest to face the bolster as you turn your head in the same direction as your knees. Place your arms on either side of the bolster with your hands over your head. Make any small adjustments to create equanimity and ease.

DIRECTION OF MOVEMENT

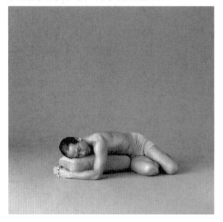

As your legs anchor you to the ground, allow your pelvis and your spine to begin to spiral into a twist. Your lower back will be especially broad in this posture—bring your breath and attention there. It's important to adjust your spine periodically to bring length to the side of your body that is lying on the bolster. The bolster supports you physically and mentally, giving you the relief of a promised nap.

Surrender into relaxation and a meditation on your breath. Extend your exhalation as you fall more completely, falling, falling, falling. . . . *The silence at the bottom of your exhalations and the settling in of your body-mind.*

ALTERNATE VIEW

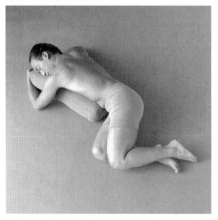

If you stay in this pose for an extended period of time, we suggest changing the position of your head as your intuition leads you. You might be surprised at what a striking difference the various positions of your head can make. Even if a single position feels very comfortable, you should still change it periodically. You often will not realize the intensity of this pose until you come out of it. Therefore we suggest that you start with the minimum amount of time in this pose, and build up your timing gradually from there. *Gentle twist, body unraveling, deep contentment.*

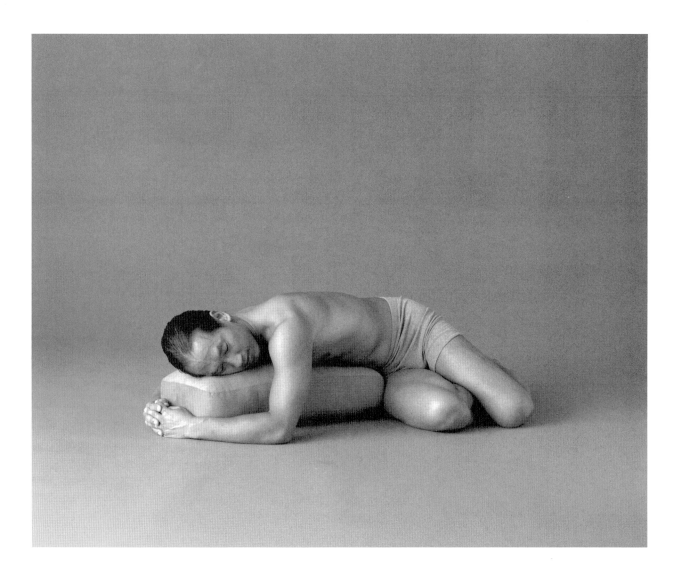

One Thing. Allow the sheer position of your body in this pose to cleanse and restore your body.

Yoga is sensual at the deepest root of sensuality—the manifestation of the human body with the breath.

Reclined Cobbler's Pose

Supta Baddha Konasana / 1 to 5 minutes

DIRECTION OF MOVEMENT

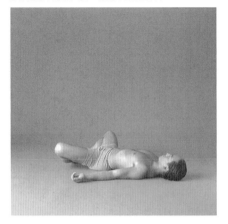

Start by lying on your back with your legs bent and the soles of your feet on the ground close to your hips. Drop your legs open so the soles of your feet come together. Position your arms on the ground so your hands are six to eight inches from your body with palms facing upward. Now turn your shoulder blades so they move farther downward toward your pelvis, and widen out from the center of your spine. This pose leaves you exposed and vulnerable yet deeply connected to earth. Give in completely, letting go of your instinctual fears, your legs gradually unfolding like Chinese tea leaves unfurling in a tea bowl, releasing their exquisite flavor.

MODIFICATION 1

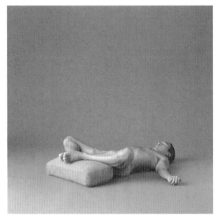

If your lower back becomes sensitive when you lie on the ground in this pose, make yourself more comfortable by placing your feet on a bolster or folded blanket. Experiment with the height of the blanket to see what brings maximum length and relief to your lower back. Know, however, that this position may also become uncomfortable if you stay in the pose for several minutes, so support your knees as well (see Modification 2). Sometimes it is more beneficial not to feel a stretch but to support yourself for maximum comfort. Often your body opens more completely when it feels safe and is not at its edge.

MODIFICATION 2

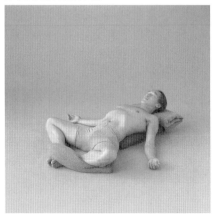

Start by placing a bolster behind you with the short edge up against your sacrum. Next take a blanket and make a long roll, and wrap the blanket roll around your feet and under your knees. Now begin to lie back on the bolster as you slightly tuck your buttocks. Then lie all the way back with your head raised slightly higher than your chest (you can use a folded blanket or towel as a pillow). Let yourself become aware of the amazing natural opening of your front body—you guard yourself so much of the time by closing it. The ecstasy that transpires from unbinding and revealing your heart feels like being deeply rooted and flying simultaneously.

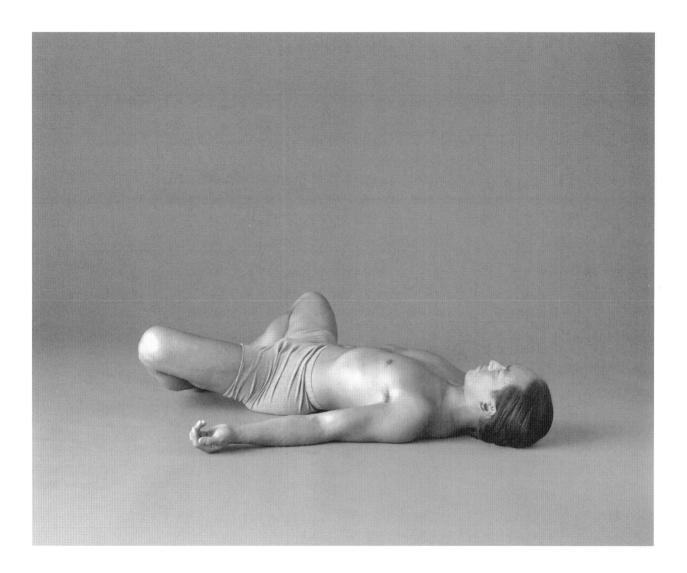

One Thing. Find the appropriate support that allows you to bathe in supreme contentment, and then turn inward to observe the subtle feelings that arise and fall.

What if you gave everything in the world the same equality—including everything in your body? What would happen? Would there be a difference between your lover and a stranger?

Legs Up the Wall Pose

Viparita Karani / 2 to 10 minutes

PREPARATION

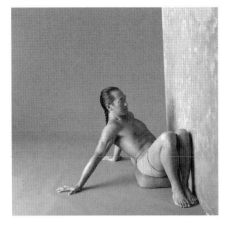

Start by putting the long edge of your bolster a couple of inches away from a wall. Then sit on the short edge of the bolster with the right side of your body against the wall. Now slowly lower yourself down on the bolster so your legs swing up the wall and your back body rests on the bolster. Adjust yourself so your shoulders rest on the ground, with the front edge of the bolster supporting your lower ribs. This should keep your chest open as your belly stays soft. Scoot yourself as close to the wall as possible, making sure your pelvis is still dropping its weight on the bolster. Extend your legs, keep them together, and press them lightly toward the wall. Make any small adjustments that will bring ease and relaxation.

DIRECTION OF MOVEMENT

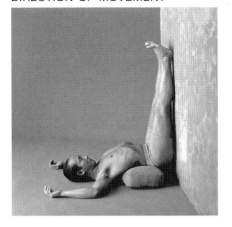

Your legs are lightly suspended, their energy and fluids cascading like a Hawaiian waterfall into the pool of your belly. *An emerald lake of quiet serenity.* Then that body of water slowly spreads into your open chest and flows into the purity of your throat, cooling and soothing your mind. Lightly press the tops of your thighs, rooting them toward the wall. As your lower back frees itself from the reins of gravity, let the harnessing of your chest be unleashed and your heart resound with its true vibrancy. Feel free to change the position of your arms to deepen your receptivity. Position your head so that your neck is in its natural curve, providing a clear conduit for energy moving along your spine.

MODIFICATION

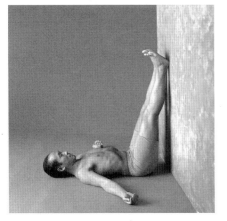

You may need to practice this pose with a bolster a number of times before your spine becomes comfortable. This position can feel foreign because so many of us have been habitually hunched forward at desks, on couches, and in cars. However, if the bolster is *too* irritating, practice this pose with your back flat on the ground. If your hamstrings are tight, move far enough away from the wall so your sacrum is supported easily by the ground. Place your arms where they feel most comfortable and where they also support the opening of the front of your chest. Allow the weight of your legs to help you surrender and release, inhale and exhale.

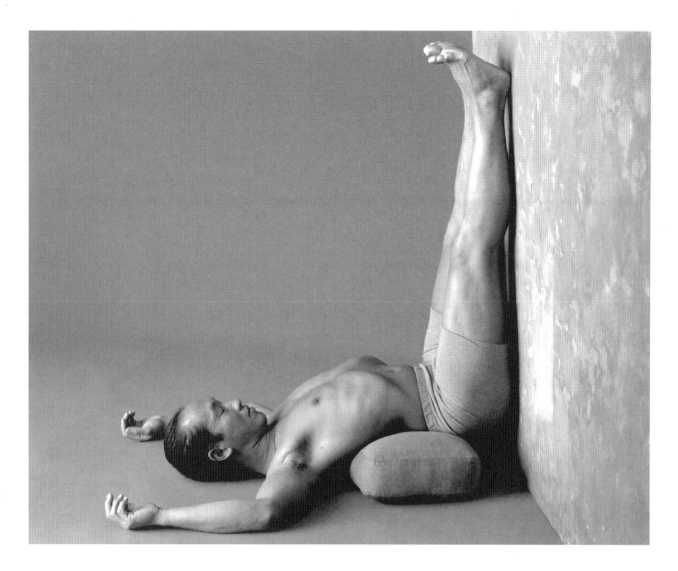

One Thing. Savor the sensation of your legs over your pelvis, your pelvis over your chest, your chest over your head—reserve a little time every day to give it all up and listen.

Lie so far back in your body that you don't know who you are. . . .

Classic Relaxation Pose

Shvanasana / 2 to 10 minutes

PREPARATION

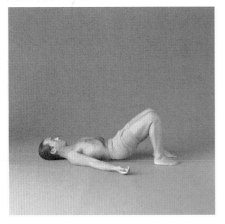

Start by lying on your back with your legs bent and the soles of your feet on the ground. Place your elbows on the ground next to your side lower ribs with your hands in the air. Now roll your shoulder blades down toward your hips as you retain a broadness between your shoulder blades. From here, lift your pelvis and slightly tuck the flesh of your buttocks toward your heels. Straighten your arms and legs along the floor with your feet about a foot apart. Rest your hands about eight inches from your hips with your palms facing upward, and let your legs and feet roll apart from each other as they relax completely.

DIRECTION OF MOVEMENT

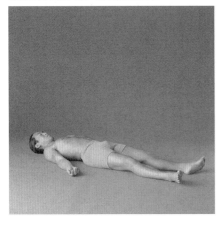

Keep your mind steady on your legs for several breaths. Notice how they begin to drop toward the ground and away from your hips. Then, for several more breaths, bring your attention to your arms and watch them as they, too, drop into the ground. As your organs of action fall slowly into nonaction, you can focus on the subtle movements of your body. Feel the beat of your heart and its pulsing echoing in the chambers of your body. Feel the rise and fall of your breath in your belly, and let that rhythm consume your consciousness. *Floating with equanimity, awareness, and surrender.*

MODIFICATION

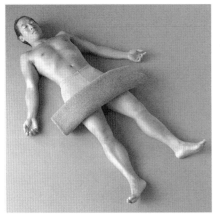

Sometimes as we lie down for Relaxation Pose, our bodies remain anxious and our minds flighty. It can be very comforting to place a folded blanket on your thighs to remind you that the letting go of your legs is an essential ingredient for calming your mind. The blanket will help you remember to breathe down into your legs and use the rhythm of your breath to caress and rock the tension out of your body. Over and over again, we bring our minds back to our legs melting into the earth.

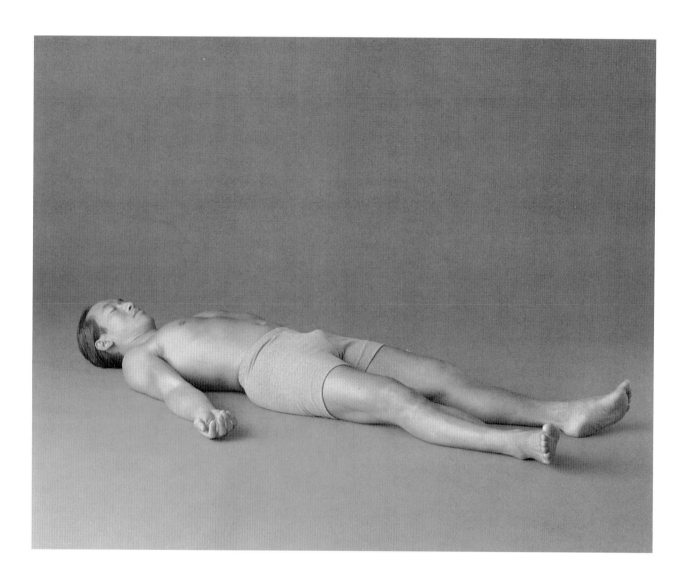

One Thing. Learning how to surrender is learning how to breathe the fragrance of life.

Listen to the wavering, the chaos of your heart.

Supported Relaxation Pose

Shavasana / 2 to 10 minutes

DIRECTION OF MOVEMENT

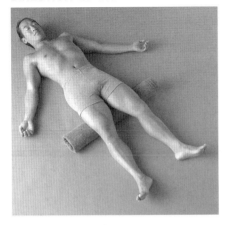

Fold a blanket into quarters and roll it into a tight roll. Place this roll under your lower thighs, close to the backs of your knees. Then lie back into Relaxation Pose and make any necessary adjustments to create ease in your back body and openness in your front body.

Drop your awareness into your back body, the muscles of your back spreading from your spine. Let the blanket roll under your legs give weight and broadness to your lower back. As your back gains more contact with the ground, relax your front body downward into that support. With your legs bent, take your inhalations into your hip joints and let your exhalations drop your thighs open onto the support of the bolster.

MODIFICATION 1

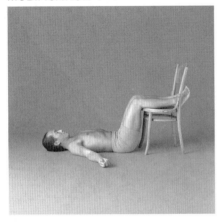

If your lower back is not comfortable with the bolster under your legs, try bringing your calves onto the seat of a chair to alleviate the pull of your legs on your spine. Tall or long-legged people may need to adjust the chair by placing blankets on the seat to find the most effective height. The beauty of this variation is that it adds a slight inversion to Relaxation Pose, which is sometimes more comforting to your nervous system. Your calf muscles spreading on the seat of the chair will facilitate a deep release because it is with these muscles that you are constantly navigating your balance. To let go in this part of your body is essential to understanding freedom from your physical habits.

MODIFICATION 2

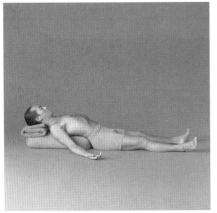

If lying with your back flat on the ground induces some physical or mental discomfort, try lying on a bolster. Start by sitting with your sacrum up against the bolster, then slowly lie down with your head on a folded blanket or pillow. Drape your arms by your sides, and move your legs slightly apart as you let them drop open. From the lift of your chest and the movement of your legs falling into the earth, your spine receives a lovely elongation. Often this variation encourages a more complete surrender, psychologically and emotionally. The openness of your heart, the grounding of your legs, and your eyes looking down and inward move you toward a silence that can break open your bindings and barriers.

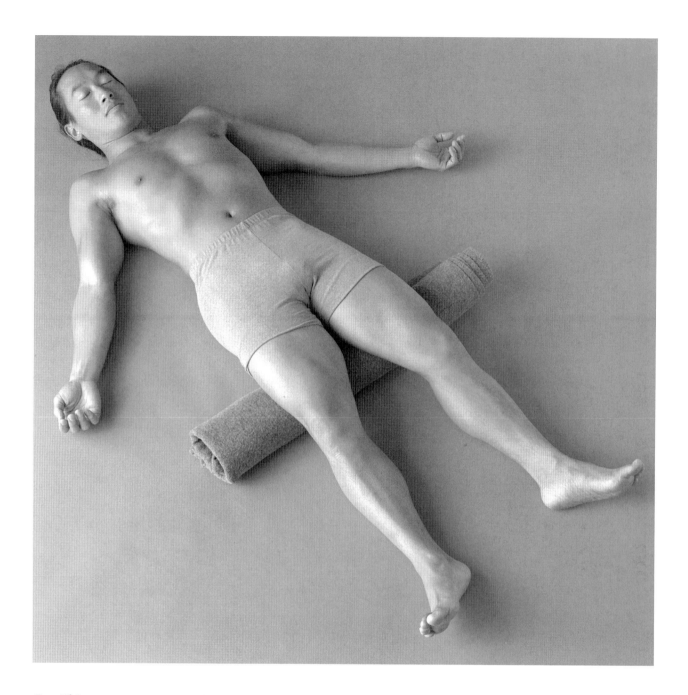

One Thing. Let your upper chest flutter with the beat of your heart, like a baby bird just out of its shell, beginning to unwrap its wings from the sticky glue of its own birth.

If nothing else, you get a little more delighted with the mystery.

Practicing at Home

ROD   Developing a home practice begins with your interest and curiosity. A lot of people are scared of starting a practice at home because they think that they don't know enough. But there's no danger in just beginning to play around with whatever knowledge you've gleaned from this book and the knowledge you have acquired over the years about your particular body and mind. Using this book, you can try different sequencing or just keep doing the eight practices. A lot of yoga is repetition. You do a lot of the same poses over and over again—daily—but what happens when you do is that you start finding new things. You realize that you can do the same postures in the same sequence and yet have a very different experience. For example, I've done Triangle Pose almost every day for twenty years, and gradually deeper and deeper subtleties have been exposed. There's an exquisite satisfaction in getting to know something that profoundly. And also, the poses work every time I've practiced. They make me feel good and enable me to be present. I get a lot out of practicing every day. I love it.

NINA   What is a good practice?

ROD   In some sense, there is no such thing as a good practice or a bad practice. There are practices that make you feel like you've accomplished something. There are practices that fill you with joy because you feel like, "Oh, I did something I've never done before!" There are practices that feel sort of crummy and sticky, like your body's not functioning very well. But the funny thing is that—usually—your body's functioning a little bit better after practice. So in some ways the practice is to check in with yourself. It's like, well, this is the way I'm feeling today; this is the way my body's feeling, and this is the way I'm thinking. Maybe you know you are moody—maybe you have PMS—and so that just gives you an idea of what you're dealing with before you go interact with the world, especially if you practice in the morning. It just gives you an idea of, for instance, oh, maybe I better take it easy today; I'm not really feeling that chipper. Or maybe I want to tackle the things at work that I've been putting off for a long time, because I'm really energetic and my mind is clear.

NINA   That all sounds really wonderful, except you often say to me, "I had a good workout this morning." You actually judge your own practices.

ROD   Yes, that's true. I'm glad you pointed that out. Sometimes I guess I judge a practice by the number of insights I get. Maybe it's like being a scientist and having an experiment reveal something. Or some new idea begins to per-colate—some new theory. And yes, that's goal-oriented, but it just happens. Maybe that's what I call a good practice, when something of interest really comes up, and it's not just a daily routine or ritual.

NINA   So that might mean that one day you might feel kind of discouraged be-cause nothing interesting came up. Like, "That wasn't so great"?

ROD   Yes. The funny thing is that after twenty years, there have been some prac-tices where nothing new comes up, nothing new and exciting, but yoga still always makes me feel better. And it's hard to deny yourself that. After you get used to feeling better, it's not that you're addicted, but it's like, well, I have this tool that makes me feel better, more clear, more able, more capa-ble.

NINA   Why don't you talk a little bit about what your practice is like.

ROD   I usually get up at five-thirty in the morning, before my family—my kids—are up. And I go into my yoga room and sit for a moment. Sometimes I start right away, and sometimes I sit around for a while in one or two poses and just wait until some intuitive notion comes up about what I want to do. Sometimes I actually have an idea the night before; I'll say, oh, tomor-row I'm going to practice back bends or forward bends. It changes all the time, what the nature of the practice is going to be.

   But anyway, my friend Ian comes over—my next-door neighbor, a classi-cal violinist—almost every day that I'm home when he's home, to practice with me. Sometimes we do the same poses in the same sequence, and sometimes we do our own things. I sometimes have other yogis and yoginis come over—students or other teachers—and we practice together, maybe on something specific that we've been wanting to work on. So it's like a yoga community that comes over. And this really helps in motivation, because if you know someone is going to be coming by, it's that much easier to get out of bed.

NINA   Do you talk to each other while you practice?

ROD   Yes, we talk to each other—we probably even talk to ourselves. Sometimes we're completely silent. Sometimes we talk about political issues, and sometimes—because Ian's a violin teacher at the conservatory in San Francisco—we talk about students and what it means to transfer knowledge to students. How students are getting it or not getting it, how you inspire them, how you teach them about some esoteric thoughts and ideas. He's talking about how to get them to perform and how to get them to hear and love music. So I'm trying to compare that with how to get people to be good teachers of yoga, how to inspire people to really look into the yoga practice, things like that. Plus, sometimes we just talk about family life. We talk about everything—current events, philosophy. We actually do talk a lot about philosophy, Ian and I. It's really my time to throw around a lot of different philosophical ideas.

NINA   The reason I wanted you to talk about this is because I know that people have a lot of angst about their own practices, and they have these ideas about the proper way to do it, that there should be a sacred space that's set up in a certain way and that needs to be totally quiet and that practicing is something that you have to do alone. I think all that sometimes gets in their way. And also that they need to practice two hours or whatever. So I think all those notions get in their way of *beginning*.

ROD   I think that's not the only thing that gets in the way. I think it's just part of human nature that to motivate oneself to do a practice—even if you love the practice—can be difficult. But this whole idea of a sacred space—I mean it's nice to have a special place in your house that has all the props, that's empty so you don't have to clear the space—it's like having an art studio when you're an artist. But in some sense the great thing about yoga is that you can practice it anywhere. I practice it in airports, in airplane seats, in offices, in hotel rooms, in the park, at the beach. I practice it with my children climbing all over me. And then sometimes I tell my kids, "Dad's off limits." It all depends what I'm doing. Some things take quiet—you can't really practice breath work when everybody's yelling. When your kids are crawling on you, you can practice some things quite well, and some things you can't. You're not going to do handstand in the middle of the room with your kids running around.

And when you're doing internal work—where you're trying to feel the subtleties of your breath and how they're affecting the posture and so forth—then it's helpful to have a quiet, open space. But my love of yoga is such that there's always some type of yoga to be done, even when you're not actually doing the postures. You can always be trying to understand the principles of yoga in every part of your life and how to apply them.

So, Nina, do you practice at home?

NINA   Yes, I do.

ROD   How often do you practice at home?

NINA   Right now I do yoga six days a week. The actual number of days I practice at home depends on how many classes I'm taking because I don't usually practice at home on the day I take a class. So generally about four times a week.

ROD   Do you remember when you first practiced at home?

NINA   I started practicing at home regularly after my first retreat with you. There were a lot of poses I couldn't do, and I felt sort of humiliated by that. I think of myself as this small, not very strong woman, and most of those poses I couldn't do had to do with arm strength—they were Push-up Pose, hand-stand, and back bend. Back bend—you did something at the retreat that made me realize it was my alignment that wasn't allowing me to go up, not my arm strength—but even then, just doing one back bend was really diffi-cult and painful for me. So those were three poses that I decided I wanted to learn how to do better—poses that my regular teacher wasn't working on with me in my classes.

ROD   So basically you're telling me your motivation was humiliation. [laughs] No, I'm joking, but what I'm saying here is that you actually connected the idea of not being able to do certain poses with the idea that you just needed to practice them more. That's a really important point. I mean, that seems like a very simple connection to make, but I don't think many people actually make that connection. I think when a lot of people can't do something, they just assume that they weren't born with the gifts to make them be able to do that, and so they just scratch that one off the list.

And it's funny, because a lot of people also tell me, "Oh, I remember I could do that when I was a kid," like a back bend, for instance. They haven't done it for years, and their body remembers doing it, but they're actually a little bit timid and scared. I think that's another thing that comes up in home practice—people are actually scared to do something that they haven't done in a long time. They're scared to hurt themselves, because, I guess, their body remembers that they've been injured before, and now, as an adult, they want to feel good, but they're not necessarily willing to risk feeling bad to feel good.

NINA   I told you recently about how I go into cold water—remember, some people dive right in, and some people don't go in at all, but I ease myself in very gradually. That's exactly how I learned to do the poses I couldn't do. I found ways of moving toward them without just struggling to do the final pose. For example, for Push-up Pose, one of my teachers showed me that I could do it with blocks under my hands. So I did that for a while until I got stronger. Then I took the blocks away. She called the blocks training wheels—"Use training wheels for a while," she said—which I loved. So actually, that's how I dealt with the fear and doubt—what you said stops people from doing things because they think they can't do it, or—

ROD   Yes, they just don't even imagine themselves doing it, or they did it before and they don't do it now because they're afraid they'll injure themselves. So sometimes there's fear of injury, and sometimes there's just fear of doing something wrong. But, in truth, the more you practice, you realize it's really a playful exploration—a playful exploration mixed with arduous work, with elation and with defeat. I mean it's like anything else. We all do have, in reality, some goals for ourselves, but after a while, like you said, you *practice*. You might even practice putting your feet behind your head, but it's not even so much that you're ever going to get your feet behind your head, it's just moving into that general shape with your body—it's liberating.

NINA   For me—because it's my personality—I use these little baby steps toward these things, so I don't have to throw myself off the cliff. But I think it depends on your personality—I actually do see some people in classes who just go for it—they don't feel that fear, and they just throw themselves into it. But I had to find a way to work with my particular personality.

ROD   That's great to know. As a teacher, one has to try to figure out what is actually going to work for someone. I mean, you might tell one person, "Just go up," and you might tell another person, "Try this, try that." There are so many different ways to approach the practice. And I think one should have fun with approaching it in different ways. I think sometimes for a person like you it's important to just go for it—just for the heck of it—just for literally not always taking baby steps—and then other times take the baby steps. I think for someone who can naturally do things already, it's actually more difficult to understand the postures. So for them, to go backward and do the little steps along the way makes them come to a deeper understanding instead of just some natural ability or natural courage that they may already have. How you approach something is very important. And taking baby steps toward a goal is actually a very intelligent way of working.

NINA   The other thing about my practice was that I began very modestly. I had those three things that I wanted to do. So I didn't say, "Oh, I have to practice for two hours," which I can do now—happily. But I didn't try to do that in the beginning. I mean, that's such a burden, if you say, "Oh, I have to practice for two hours"—then you can't find the time or the motivation. So I just started by doing those poses. And then the practice grew up around that. Because, well, if you do a back bend, you need to do something to warm up beforehand and you need to do something for your back afterward. So actually, it was almost comical. It kept getting longer and longer—because I just kept throwing this in and throwing that in. But it did evolve in a very organic way. For instance, I did Sun Salutations around the Push-up Pose, and that type of thing.

ROD   Right. So give us an approximation of how much time you actually started with. You say maybe now you can practice for two hours because you want to and because it feels good, but how much time did you start with, approximately, in the beginning?

NINA   In the beginning it was often a really small amount of time, say, fifteen or twenty minutes. Maybe some days I just worked on my handstand, and I just did two handstands. One of the things I like to say to people who ask me about how I started my practice—people who say, "I wish I could practice like you"—is "Change your clothes." And they look at me oddly and ask, "What do you mean, change my clothes?" And I say, "Well, you know, just go put on some yoga clothes, and then once you're in your yoga clothes, you're going to have to do something, right? Because you went to all the trouble to change your clothes." From my experience, that's how it was. I changed my clothes, and I did handstand or whatever, and it grew out of that.

ROD   We have so many social postures. And specific postures go with specific clothes. For instance, when you go to the opera, you dress up, and when you go running, you wear workout clothes. Most of us become somewhat bound by these conventions. If we know this about ourselves, then it's important either to change your clothes or to change your identifications with the clothes you have on. For instance, why not do Triangle Pose in your office in a business suit? Why not kick up into handstand at the airport?

NINA For me, it was more of a psychological trick than a feeling that I couldn't do yoga in my everyday clothes. It was more like a little ritual that kicked off the whole practice.

ROD That sounds like the story one of my friends tells—he says he sets his clock at nighttime so that he'll go to sleep on time. That way he'll wake up in the morning and feel ready to practice before work. So his practice of yoga actually starts the night before. His clock goes off at nine o'clock, and he knows, whatever social situation he's in, it's time to leave. And then he goes home, does a little reading, gets in bed, and is in bed at a certain time, and then he wakes up early to do his practice. So it's interesting—yes, "Go change your clothes." Maybe just throw yourself in a handstand no matter where you are. My friend used to do a hundred handstands a day just because he wanted to learn it, and he'd kick up onto every wall he saw. Yes—don't let your mind or anything get in the way. Just *begin*.

PART 6

Unwrapping It

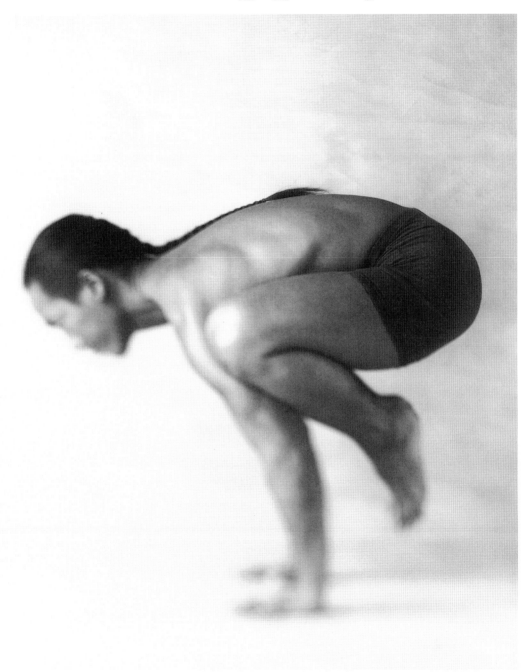

Winter solitude—
in a world of one color
the sound of wind.

— BASHŌ

So here we are at the end of the book. Maybe some of you have done the practices, while others of you have read the dialogues. Maybe some of you do yoga every day, while others of you do yoga once a month. And Nina wants me to come up with some kind of conclusion for you, some ending to the book that will "wrap things up."

But if there's one thing I've learned in all these years of yoga, it's that when you inquire deeply into anything, you're basically left with a bunch of confusion and conflicting answers. And I don't necessarily think that's ever going to clear up. When I listen to myself in my yoga practice, I feel all kinds of different impulses. I think, let's see, I've got to go pick up the kids today, I've got to go teach today, and I've got a phone interview at ten, or oh, I haven't seen my parents for a while and they're probably going to die soon, and my kids are growing up—how many more times will they sit in my lap?—maybe I need to cut my schedule back, or oh, is it really that interesting to pay so much attention to my body?—maybe I should just go take a walk, or oh, how much of what I'm holding up is really worth *anything?* or God, just sitting here listening to my breath is so soothing, it feels like ointment on a burn. You know, you start hearing all these voices, and it's actually just

a bunch of chatter. So you start wondering, where is all the chatter going? Where are all my wants, desires, expectations, and thoughts leading me? Obviously, it's led you—all the chattering, difficulty, clarity, and confusion—to sitting right here with this book, in this very moment in time. And for me, yoga simply means continuing to be with *what is* and allowing that to be a crazy, chaotic mess. So isn't it impossible to have a nice clean ending to this book?

But most of us aren't very comfortable with that. We want to wrap everything up in a clean little package, tie the bow on it, put the Scotch tape in the right places, and make the folds all nice and neat, and then send it away. But then it goes to the post office and it gets all messed up anyway. I know that when people read this book, they're going to have different interpretations of what I've said. And then when we meet on the street, we'll probably argue about it! But that's going to be wonderful. We just can't take it all that seriously.

Because you want to learn something about yoga, I've been showing you a little of what I think it's about. But I don't know where this practice is leading me. I don't know what I'm doing with it. I don't know what I'm going to find. I just keep on scratching around, and sniffing around, and looking for another bone to dig up. And as far as I can see, that just means reoccurring inquisitiveness, reoccurring boredom, reoccurring enlightenment, and reoccurring frustration.

What is coming out of the yoga practice for me is being able to savor something more completely—this thing called *living*. It's like wanting a toy for Christmas. When I was a kid, I really wanted a race car set, and I never got it. I got other things for Christmas instead, so what was I going to do? Cry and be frustrated that I didn't get a race car set? Well, yes, that's exactly what I did, and wish for one next Christmas, again and again, and I never got one. I did get other things, and I did enjoy other things, but it wasn't the end of the story of my unquenched thirst for a race car set. Now I can buy one for myself, but I haven't done it. Because if yoga has done anything for me, it's allowed me to see this joke about myself—my desire and the fulfillment or lack of fulfillment of it, and then a new desire. Suffering and then alleviation of the suffering, and then more suffering and the alleviation of that suffering. The boredom. The excitement. I'm beginning to think, oh, different colors. Fall colors, spring colors, winter colors, summer colors. Am I going to have a preference? Am I going to keep on wanting some things and pushing some things away? It has happened to me enough times that I'm starting to have an internal laugh going on. Actually, it's funny *and* it's sad. I've come to a place where I feel like laughing and crying every moment of the day.

So I feel like there just is *no ending*. And you know that uneasy feeling that you're left with when things don't wrap themselves up—like when you read a book or see a movie that has a final scene where absolutely *nothing* gets resolved—that's the feeling you started with. And you know the feeling that's churning your gut and making you do all kinds of weird things in the world? That feeling is still here. We could wrap everything up in this book, so you would feel a sense of relief—oh, good, that feeling is gone, because everything is sewn up in a perfect little circle. But that would only last until you started to bleed again.

So should we end with an illusion? Or should we end with that never-ceasing difficulty and say, oh, there it is again—it hurts?

Appendix A

Resources

Rodney's Personal, Idiosyncratic Reading Recommendations

Light on Pranayama: The Yogic Art of Breathing. By B. K. S. Iyengar. New York: Crossroad Publishing Company, 1985.

Light on Yoga. By B. K. S. Iyengar. New York: Schocken, 1995.

The Heart of Yoga: Developing a Personal Practice. By T. K. V. Desikachar. Rochester, Vt.: Inner Traditions International, 1999.

Being Peace. By Thich Nhat Hanh. Berkeley, Calif.: Parallax Press, 1926, 1996.

When Things Fall Apart: Heart Advice for Difficult Times. By Pema Chodron. Boston: Shambhala Publications, 1999.

Cutting Through Spiritual Materialism. By Chogyam Trungpa. Boston: Shambhala Publications, 1939, 1987.

The Essential Rumi. By Jelalludin Rumi. Translated by Coleman Barks. New York: Harper Trade, 1997.

The Gift: Poems by Hafiz the Great Sufi Master. By Hafiz of Shiraz. Translated by Daniel Ladinsky. New York: Viking Penguin, 1999.

Otherwise: New and Selected Poems. By Jane Kenyon. Saint Paul, Minn.: Graywolf Press, 1997.

A Book of Luminous Things. Edited by Czeslaw Milosz. San Diego: Harcourt, 1998.

On Fear. By Jiddhu Khrishnamurti. San Francisco: Harper San Francisco, 1895, 1986.

Think on These Things. By Jiddhu Khrishnamurti. New York: Harper Trade, 1895, 1986.

Videos

Yoga Videos with Rodney Yee
Abs Yoga for Beginners (30 minutes)

AM Yoga for Beginners (30 minutes)

Art of Breath and Relaxation (60 minutes) (also available as audio)

Back Care Yoga for Beginners (30 minutes)

Power Yoga for Beginners—Flexibility (30 minutes)

Power Yoga for Beginners—Stamina (30 minutes)

Power Yoga for Beginners—Strength (30 minutes)

Upper Body Yoga for Beginners (30 minutes)

Yoga Conditioning for Athletes (60 minutes)

Yoga for Meditation (75 minutes)

Yoga for Relaxation (75 minutes)

Yoga for Two for Beginners (30 minutes)

Yoga Practice for Energy (60 minutes)

Yoga Practice for Intermediates (70 minutes)

Yoga Practice for Strength (75 minutes)

Yoga Remedies for Natural Healing (60 minutes)

Other Living Arts Videos

Lower Body Yoga for Beginners with Suzanne Deason (30 minutes)

PM Yoga for Beginners with Patricia Walden (30 minutes)

Stress Relief Yoga with Suzanne Deason (30 minutes)

Yoga Practice: Introduction with Patricia Walden (70 minutes)

Yoga Practice for Beginners with Patricia Walden (75 minutes)

Yoga Practice for Flexibility with Patricia Walden (80 minutes)

Yoga Remedies for Balance with Suzanne Deason (60 minutes)

Yoga Props (and Clothes) by Mail

Living Arts Catalog
360 Interlocken Blvd., Suite 300
Broomfield, CO 80021-3492
Phone: 800-254-8464
FAX: 800-582-6872
Web site: www.gaiam.com

Tools for Yoga Prop Shop and Mail Order Catalogue
2 Green Village Road
Madison, NJ 07940
Phone: 888-678-9642 (U.S. and Canada) or 973-966-5311
FAX: 800-310-9833
Web site: www.yogapropshop.com

Finding a Yoga Teacher

Yoga Journal's Source 2001 Annual Guide
2054 University Avenue, Suite 600
Berkeley, CA 94704
Phone: 510-841-9200
FAX: 510-644-3101
Web site: www.yogajournal.com

Yoga International Magazine's Yoga Teacher's Guide
Online only: www.yogateachersguide.org

Retreats and Workshops

For information about Rodney Yee's retreats and workshops around the country and abroad, see his web site: www.yeeyoga.com
Or contact: Piedmont Yoga Studio
P.O. Box 11458
Oakland, CA 94611
Phone: 510-536-8960
Email: pys@piedmontyoga.com

Contacting the Authors

Rodney Yee
c/o Piedmont Yoga Studio
P.O. Box 11458
Oakland, CA 94611
Email: rodney@yeeyoga.com

Nina Zolotow
c/o Piedmont Yoga Studio
P.O. Box 11458
Oakland, CA 94611
Email: nina@wanderingmind.com
For information about Nina's one-sentence stories, see: www.wanderingmind.com

Appendix B

Yoga and Watermelons

Watermelons have a lot to say about yoga—and about your life—if you know how to listen to them. It is as simple as this:

1. Purchase a very large, ripe watermelon. (To test for ripeness, thump briskly on the rind and listen for that lovely resonance—you'll recognize it when you hear it because it just sounds so *right*.)
2. Take the watermelon home, and then, carrying the melon, walk outside and stand on any open patch of pavement, cement, or bricks (your patio, the sidewalk, whatever).
3. On a deep inhalation, lift the watermelon over your head.
4. Exhale, and feel the alignment of your entire body under the watermelon.
5. Take a long, smooth inhalation as you ground your feet, and then, on your exhalation, throw the watermelon onto the pavement as strongly as you can, using your whole body, with complete conviction.
6. Contemplate the beauty of the smashed melon—the passionate red of its flesh, the tender white of its inner rind, the exquisite asymmetry of the jagged cracks in its green shell.
7. Now squat down on the pavement and try to put the watermelon back together.
8. . . .
9. Oh, never mind. Get the kids, call some friends, invite the neighbors, and then have everyone just dig in. Maybe even sprinkle the watermelon with a few grains of salt.
10. *Namaste.**

*A Sanskrit term of greeting, traditionally used to end a yoga class. A rough translation is, "I salute your soul."

Permissions

Grateful acknowledgment is given for permission to reprint the following poems from:

Index

Yoga poses (in English and Sanskrit) appear in regular and small capital letters.

BOW POSE
    in Breath Practice, 114
    detailed description and photos,
        276–77
    mentioned, 48
    Sanskrit term: Dhanurasana
breath, the
    counting, in order to time poses,
        30
    exercises in observing, 192–202
    following, 124
    observing the, 111, 118, 147,
        191–93, 208
    riding, 166
Breath Games, 194–202
Breathing, 119
breathing, 111
Breathing on Your Belly, in Playful
    Practice, 36
Breath Practice, 30, 109–20
    summary (photo sequence), 120
BRIDGE POSE
    See also SUPPORTED BRIDGE POSE
        in Alignment Practice, 97
    detailed description and photos,
        280–81
    related to other poses, 98
    Sanskrit term: Setu Bandha
        Sarvangasana

calf, 8, 11
CAT POSE
    detailed description and photos,
        224–25
    in Playful Practice, 37
    Sanskrit term: Chakravakasana
centering, 55, 91
CHAKRAVAKASANA. *See* CAT POSE
change, personal, 184–86
CHATURANGA DANDASANA. *See*
    PUSH-UP POSE
chest, 11
"Children pretending to be
    cormorants" (Issa), 33
CHILD'S POSE
    See also SUPPORTED CHILD'S POSE

detailed description and photos,
    296–97
in Playful Practice, 38
related to other poses, 226
Sanskrit term: Balasana
City of My Youth (Milosz), 165
clothes, yoga, 12–13, 326–27,
    334
Coat, The (Yeats), 2
Cobbler's Forward Bend, in
    Resistance Practice, 131
COBBLER'S POSE
    detailed description and photos,
        290–91
    in Grounding Practice, 74
    mentioned, 10
    related to other poses, 100
    Sanskrit term: Baddha Konasana
COBRA
    in Breath Practice, 113
    detailed description and photos,
        270–71
    in Resistance Practice, 135
    Sanskrit term: Bhujangasana
collarbones, 10
communal life, 163
Completing Your Exhalations
    (game), 198
connectedness to the earth, 77
counting breaths, 30
Cremation (Jeffers), 6
Crossed-Legged Forward Bend
    with bolster, 152
    detailed description and photos,
        298–99
    in Relaxation Practice, 152
crown of head, 11

DANDASANA. *See* STAFF POSE
death, 107–8, 147
defending one's point of view,
    206–7
depth of yoga practice, 111
desire, 332
DHANURASANA. *See* BOW POSE
Dickenson, Emily, xvii

difficult poses, 138, 161–62, 211
    and life's difficulties, 130
Directing Your Inhalation (game),
    197
Direction of Your Breath (game),
    195–96
DOWNWARD-FACING DOG
    in Alignment Practice, 96
    detailed description and photos,
        226–27
    in Falling Practice, 58
    in Grounding Practice, 71
    mentioned, 12, 20, 50, 90
    in Playful Practice, 39
    related to other poses, 272
    in Sun Salutation, 172, 175
    Sanskrit term: Adho Mukha
        Shvanasana

ego, 162
emotions, 105–6
    balanced, 185
    creating, with yoga poses, 145
exhaling, 112, 196
EXTENDED STANDING FORWARD
    BEND
    detailed description and photos,
        236–37
    in Movement Practice, 167
    in Sun Salutation, 171, 172, 176
    Sanskrit term: Uttanasana
eye pillow, 17

falling, 55
falling asleep, 30–31
Falling Practice, 30, 53–66
    mentioned, 47
    summary (photo sequence), 64
fathering, 143–44
fear, 142–43
feet, 7–8
    bare, 12, 77
First River, 179
flexibility, 49
following
    breath, 124

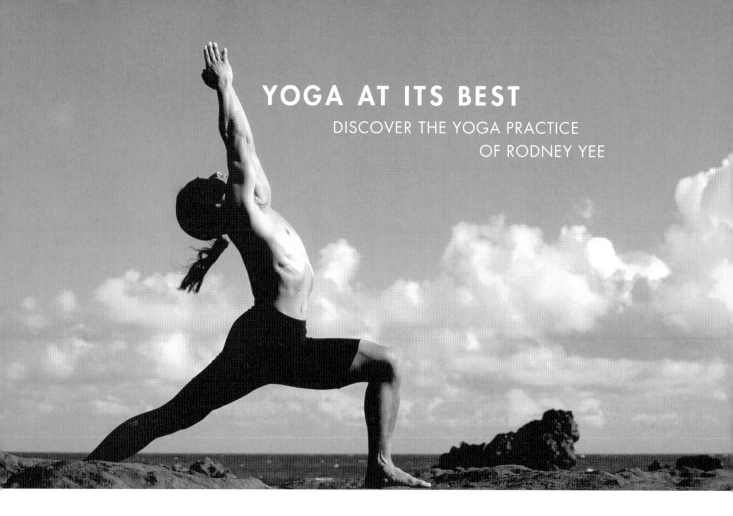
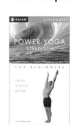
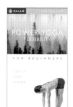
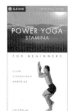
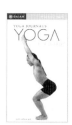
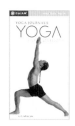
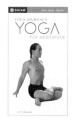
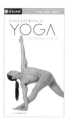
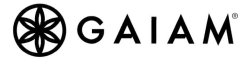